GLUTEN-FREE TRAVEL IN JAPAN

Penny Farrant

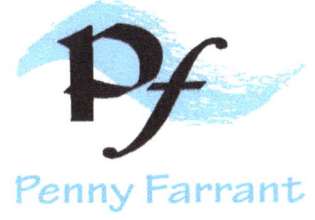

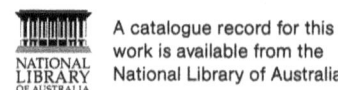

A catalogue record for this work is available from the National Library of Australia

GLUTEN-FREE TRAVEL IN JAPAN
by Penny Farrant

© 2021, PENNY FARRANT, PERTH, AUSTRALIA

All rights reserved. No part of this book may be reproduced, stored in a retrieval system, or transmitted in any form or by any means, electronic, mechanical, recording or otherwise, without the prior written permission of the author and copyright holder.

The information, views, opinions and visuals expressed in this publication are the sole expression and opinion of its author.

This book is not intended to be a substitute for medical advice from a fully qualified medical practitioner. The reader should consult with their doctor in any matters relating to his/her health.

TEXT: Penny Farrant

PHOTOGRAPHS: Penny Farrant

ISBN: 978-0-6485088-1-6 (paperback)

PUBLISHER: Penny Farrant; for special orders email: pennyfarrant@gmail.com

BISAC CODES: Travel, Asia East, Japan TRV003050; ; Health & Fitness, Allergies HEA027000

COVER PHOTO: Japanese style breakfast prepared at the Guest House Asora, Aso Town, Kyushu.

ACKNOWLEDGMENTS: Special thanks to Diana Iles for proof-reading and providing invaluable feedback & Helen Iles (Linellin Press WA) for publishing advice.

Contents

INTRODUCTION 5

1. **Coeliac disease** — *Coeliac disease, genetics & gluten-free diet* 9
2. **Planning your trip** — *Where to go, where to stay & what to do* 13
3. **Tours & walks** — *Communicating dietary requirements* 17
4. **Cooking classes** — *Japanese meals, sushi & noodles* 21
5. **Hotels** — *Breakfasts, lunches and dinners & eating in* 25
6. **Other accommodation** — *Ryokans, Airbnbs, pensions, hostels & Youth Hostels* 29
7. **Japanese cuisine** — *Restaurants, teishoku, izakaya, barbecue & nabe* 33
8. **Other cuisines** — *Indian, Thai, Italian, Spanish & others* 37
9. **Takeaways** — *Convenience stores, supermarkets & railway stations* 41
10. **Snacks** — *Nibbles & snack foods* 45
11. **Venues & events** — *Tourist venues, festivals & street foods, Christmas & New Year* 49
12. **Cooking at home** — *Kitchen appliances, utensils, crockery & cutlery* 53
13. **Meals at home** — *Breakfasts, lunches & dinners* 57
14. **Shopping for ingredients** — *Department stores, supermarkets & growers' markets* 61
15. **Fruit & vegetables** — *What's available and where to buy* 65
16. **Seafood, meat, tofu, eggs & dairy** — *What's available and where to buy* 69
17. **Mochi, sweets, cakes, desserts & icecreams** — *What's available and where to buy* 73
18. **Alcoholic drinks** — *Beer, sake, wine & spirits* 77
19. **Non-alcoholic drinks** — *Tea, coffee, chocolate & other drinks* 81
20. **Gluten-free highlights in Hokkaido** — *Wakkanai, Niseko, Sapporo & Kushiro* 85
21. **Gluten-free highlights in Honshu** — *Saitama, Takayama Nikko, Nagano & Tazawako* 89
22. **Gluten-free highlights in Shikoku** — *Naoshima, Matsuyama, Uchiko, Kochi & Sukumo* 93
23. **Gluten-free highlights in Kyushu** — *Fukuoka, Aso Town, Kagoshma & Yakushima* 97
24. **Gluten-free highlights in Okinawa** — *Itoman, Naha & Ishigaki* 101

Practical tips & advice 106

INDEX 108

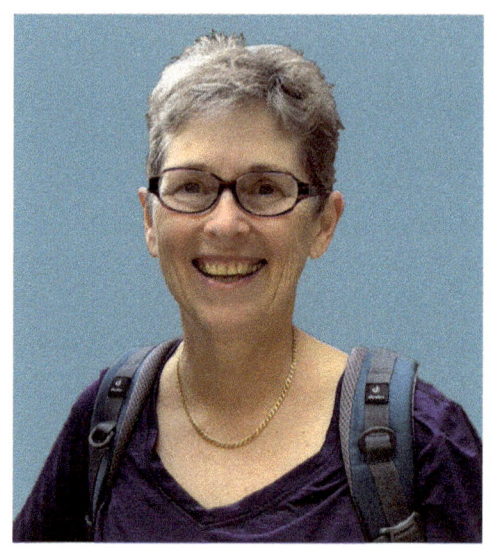

ABOUT THE AUTHOR:

Dr Penny (Penelope) Farrant was born in Melbourne, Victoria but lived most of her life in Sydney, New South Wales, where she retired in 2015 before moving to Perth, Western Australia, in 2019. She has degrees in architecture and marine biology and is particularly interested in the art-science interface. She is the author of *Colour in Nature — a Visual and Scientific Exploration* (Blandford UK 1997) and *Pen-Pen's Journey* (Vivid Publishing Fremantle WA 2016). Her interests include art and calligraphy, swimming, bushwalking and travel.

Penny and her husband Bill have visited Japan three times. They first visited Japan for five weeks in 1991–1992, at which time they fell in love with the country and made a plan to return for an entire year after they retired. They took up the challenge and spent a year in Japan in 2016–2017. By that stage Bill had been diagnosed with coeliac disease, so he faced the additional challenge of having to avoid foods containing wheat, barley, rye and oats. As seniors on a limited budget, and despite Bill having coeliac disease, they spent a rewarding year in Japan meeting many of the locals, learning about Japanese culture, sampling a range of interesting and delicious foods, and enjoying a wealth of remarkable and exciting experiences. They returned to Japan for three months in 2018 and intend to visit again.

Penny sent a weekly email to friends during their year away, with photos and descriptions of their experiences. Those emails form the basis of both this and her accompanying book *Budget Travel in Japan*, which describes their adventures week-by-week during that year in Japan.

INTRODUCTION

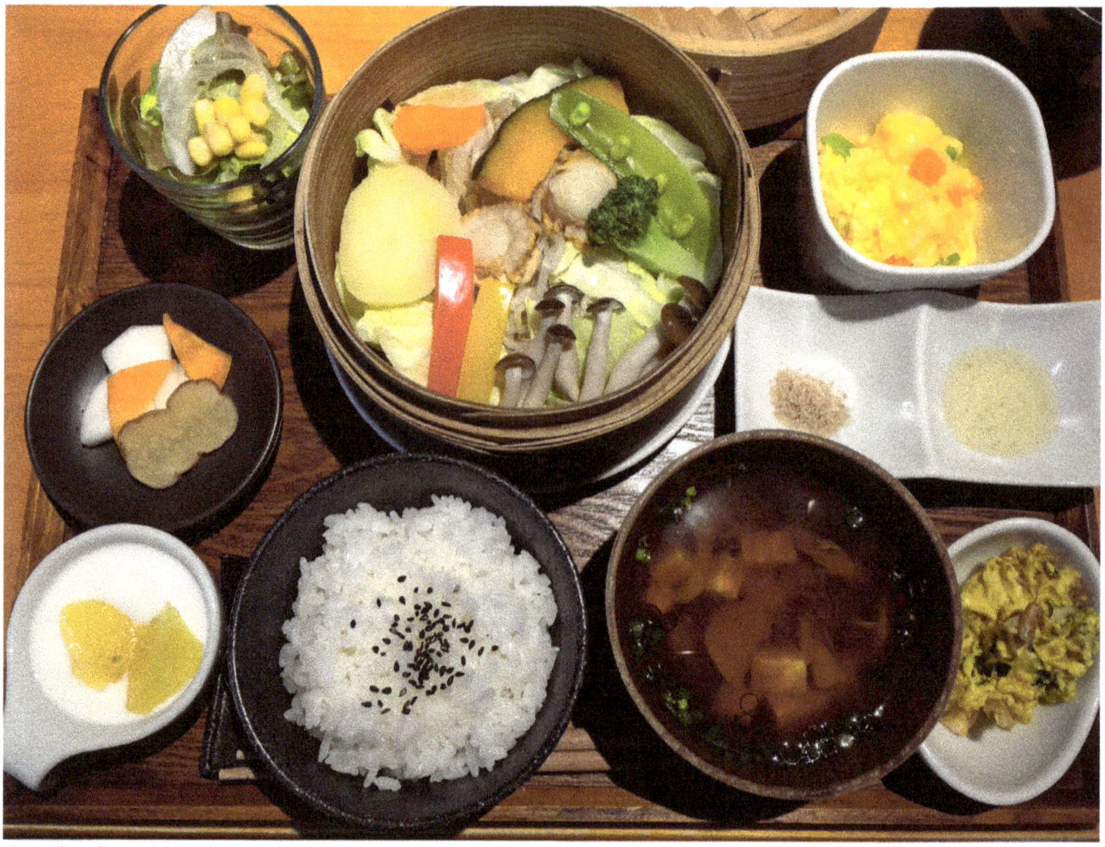

Above: Gluten-free meal, Tazawako; Row Below: Mochi packet; pink box states 'made in a factory with other products containing egg, wheat & peanuts' (yellow = wheat)

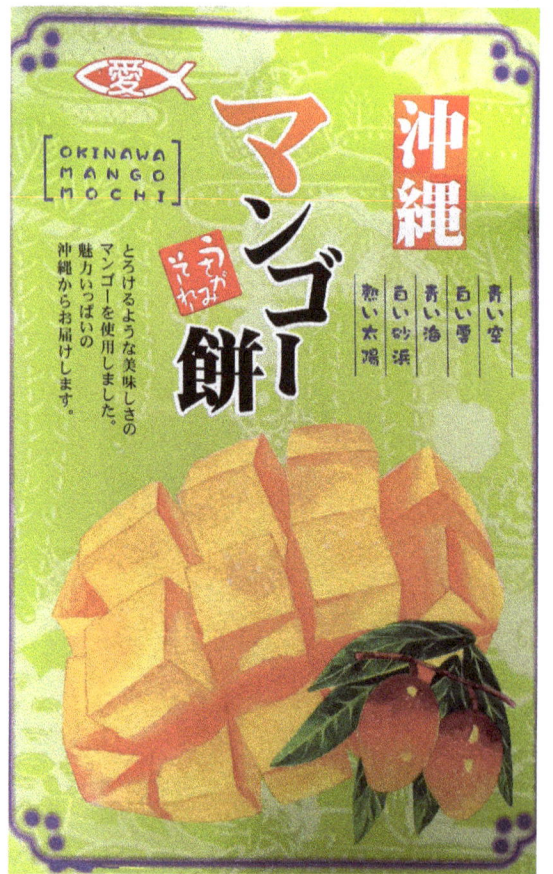

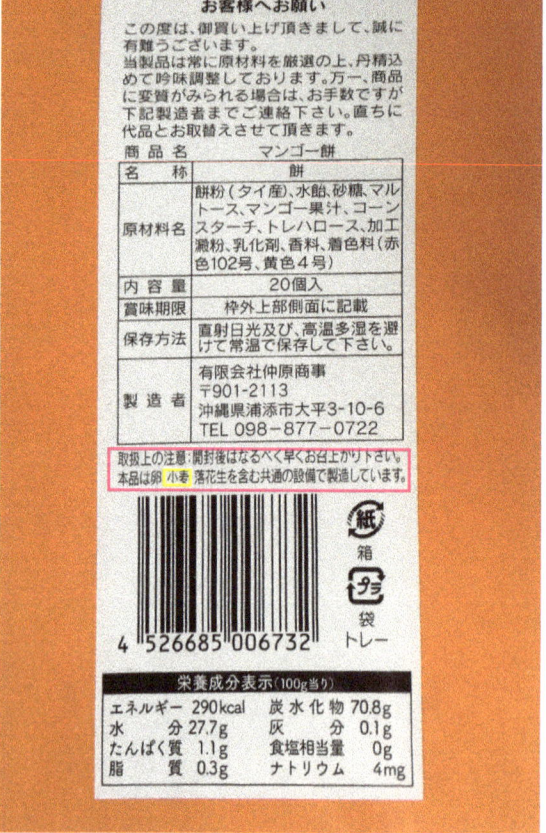

INTRODUCTION

Japan is an intriguing country, as well known for its culinary delights as its beautiful landscapes and gentle people. Yet Australians like my husband Bill who have coeliac disease (see Chapter 1) and are allergic to wheat, barley, rye and oats, are generally advised not to travel to Japan, or if they do, to expect very limited dietary options. Articles written by coeliac travellers in travel magazines usually advise other coeliacs to avoid Japan and there are few guides to inform or encourage English-speaking coeliacs to travel to Japan with confidence.

This is a shame, because Japan has a lot to offer international tourists. With a bit of planning they will find it's possible to eat well there while following a gluten-free diet and thus avoiding unwanted short- or long-term illnesses. It certainly doesn't mean that they have to eat little more than rice, fish and vegetables.

This book

After our trip to Japan in 1991–1992, my husband Bill and I made a plan to spend an entire year there after we retired. By then Bill had been diagnosed with coeliac disease, so we had to be sure that he would be able to eat well for an entire year with the prospect of gluten-free food supposedly being largely unavailable.

This book is based on our experiences during a year spent living in Japan and it complements my travel book called *Budget Travel in Japan*. *Gluten-Free Travel in Japan* tells the story of how we managed to communicate coeliac dietary requirements for tours we did, cooking classes we took, various types of accommodation we stayed at and restaurants we ate at. I also tell you about the takeaways and snacks we bought, meals we cooked ourselves using the various sorts of ingredients available, alcoholic and non-alcoholic drinks we imbibed, and the gluten-free highlights we discovered in each of the five main islands of Japan.

Fortunately Bill doesn't become ill as soon as he eats a meal containing a small amount of gluten. His symptoms are long-term, but he still needs to avoid gluten. For coeliacs with zero gluten tolerance, we urge you to choose simple dishes, be extra vigilant and not take our advice as absolute. All we can say is that Bill thrived on the food documented in this book!

Communicating dietary requirements

The Japanese language is difficult for English-speaking travellers, and the inability to communicate dietary allergies is an obstacle for people with coeliac disease who must exclude gluten from their diet in a country where gluten-free meals are rare. The low incidence of the disease in Japan means that Japanese people simply don't have a great understanding of the disease. Yet despite this, they are only too willing to help if we can communicate our needs to them.

Naturally if you travel to Japan and you are coeliac you don't want to be stuck eating a boring diet. You want the whole experience without having to learn the language! That said, if you aren't travelling with a Japanese-speaking friend, there are some important 'kanji' (characters) that you should learn to recognise, as well as a basic statement about your allergy, all of which you can read or show people by way of explanation. You can also use 'restaurant cards' to try to explain your allergy. Google Translate is useful, but only up to a point, as it isn't always accurate.

Photo Page 5: Occasionally you can find gluten-free products in Japanese supermarkets.

Coeliac disease: セリアック病 seriakku byou

Wheat: 小麦 komugi, or 小麦粉 komugiko
Barley: 麦 mugi or 大麦 oo-mugi
Rye: ライ麦 raimugi
Oats: からす麦 karasumugi
Malt: 麦芽 bakuga
Soy sauce: 醤油, shoyu
I am allergic to soy sauce and wheat: 私は醤油と小麦にアレルギーがあります
Watashi wa shōyu to komugi ni arerugī ga arimasu

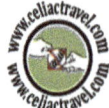

English Gluten Free Restaurant Card

I have an illness called Celiac Disease and have to follow a strict gluten free diet.

I may therefore become very ill if I eat food containing flours or grains of wheat, rye, barley and oats.

Does this food contain flour or grains of wheat, rye, barley or oats? If you are at all uncertain about what the food contains, please tell me.

I can eat food containing rice, maize, potatoes, all kinds of vegetables and fruit, eggs, cheese, milk, meat and fish - **as long as they are not cooked with wheat flour, batter, breadcrumbs or sauce.**

Thank you for your help.

© Copyright Celiac Travel.com

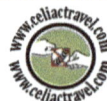

Japanese Gluten Free Restaurant Card

私はセリアック病です。厳密なグルテンフリーの食事療法に従わなくてはなりません。

小麦、ライ麦、大麦、オーツ麦、オートを含む食品を食べるとアレルギー症状をおこし、危険です。

ここで食べる食品の中に、小麦、ライ麦、大麦、オーツ麦、オートを含むものがあれば、教えて下さい。含まれているかどうか、不確かな場合も、不確かだと教えて下さい。

米、ジャガイモなどのイモ類、トウモロコシ、野菜、果物、卵、チーズ、牛乳、肉や魚は食べられます。

肉や魚の調理に小麦粉が使われていたり、小麦粉やパン粉を使った衣やソースが使われている場合は食べられません。

ご協力いただきありがとうございます。

© Copyright Celiac Travel.com

Row Above: Restaurant cards available from the Coeliac Travel website

Below: Penny and Bill at sushi class, Fukuoka — all ingredients were gluten-free

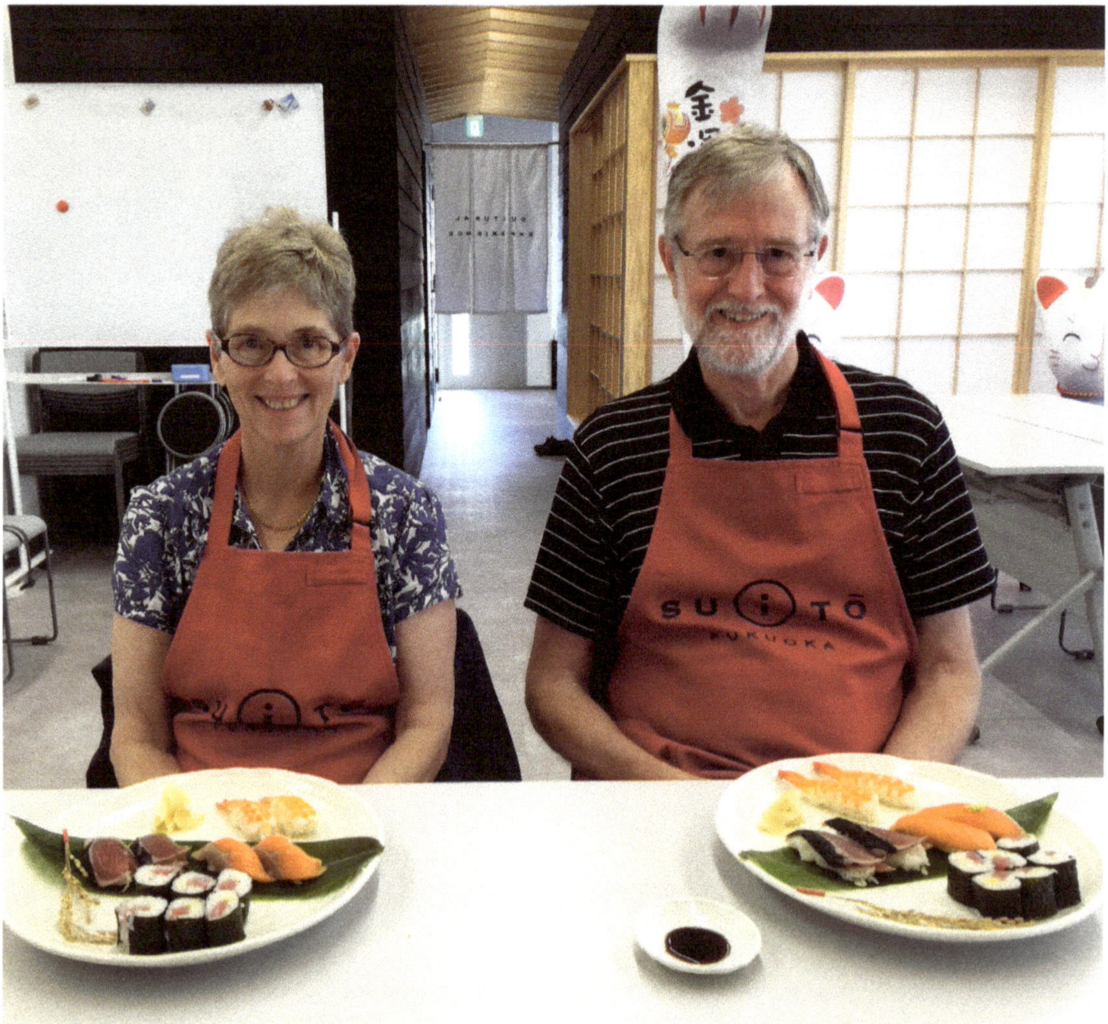

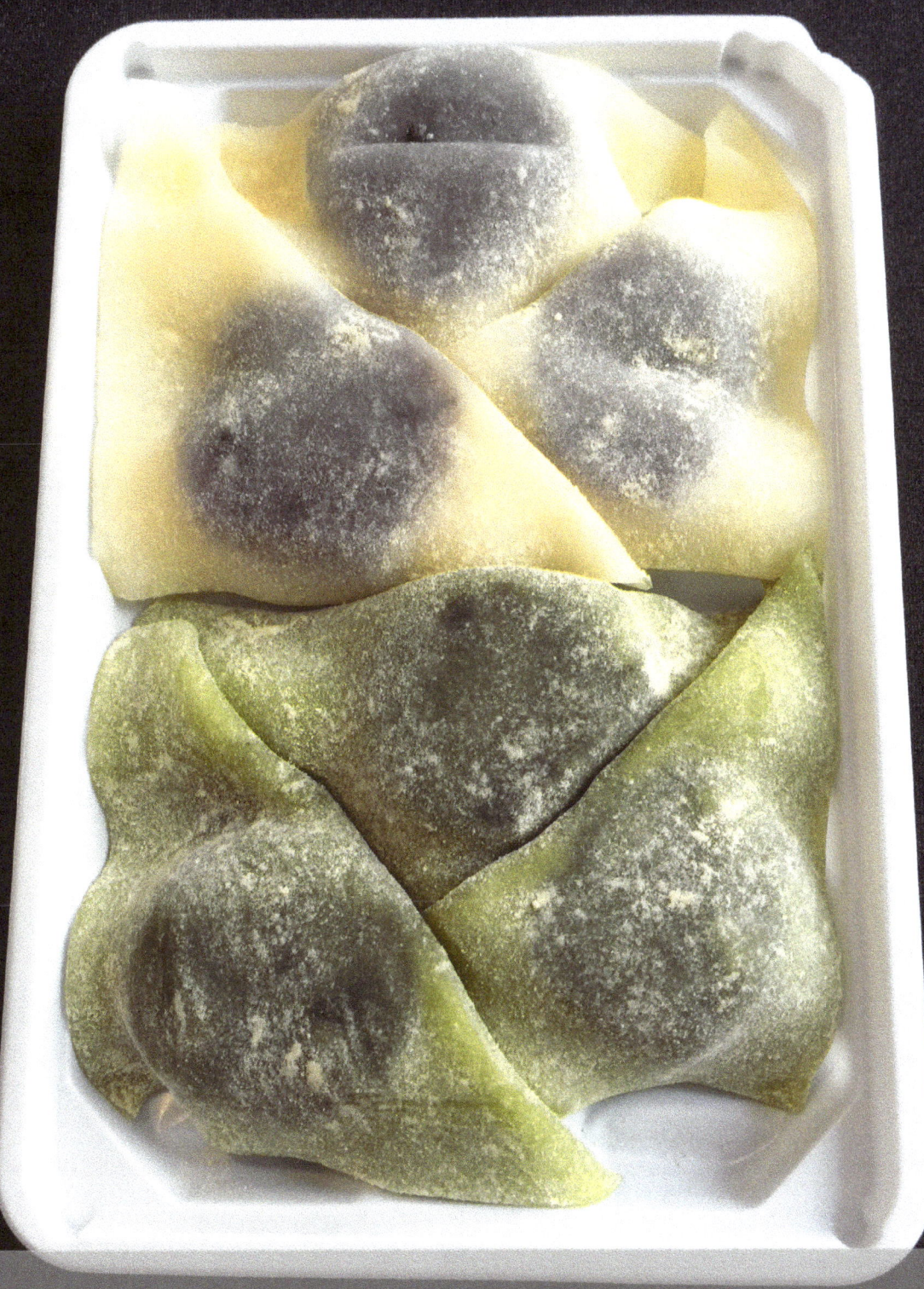

Coeliac disease
Coeliac disease, genetics & gluten-free diet

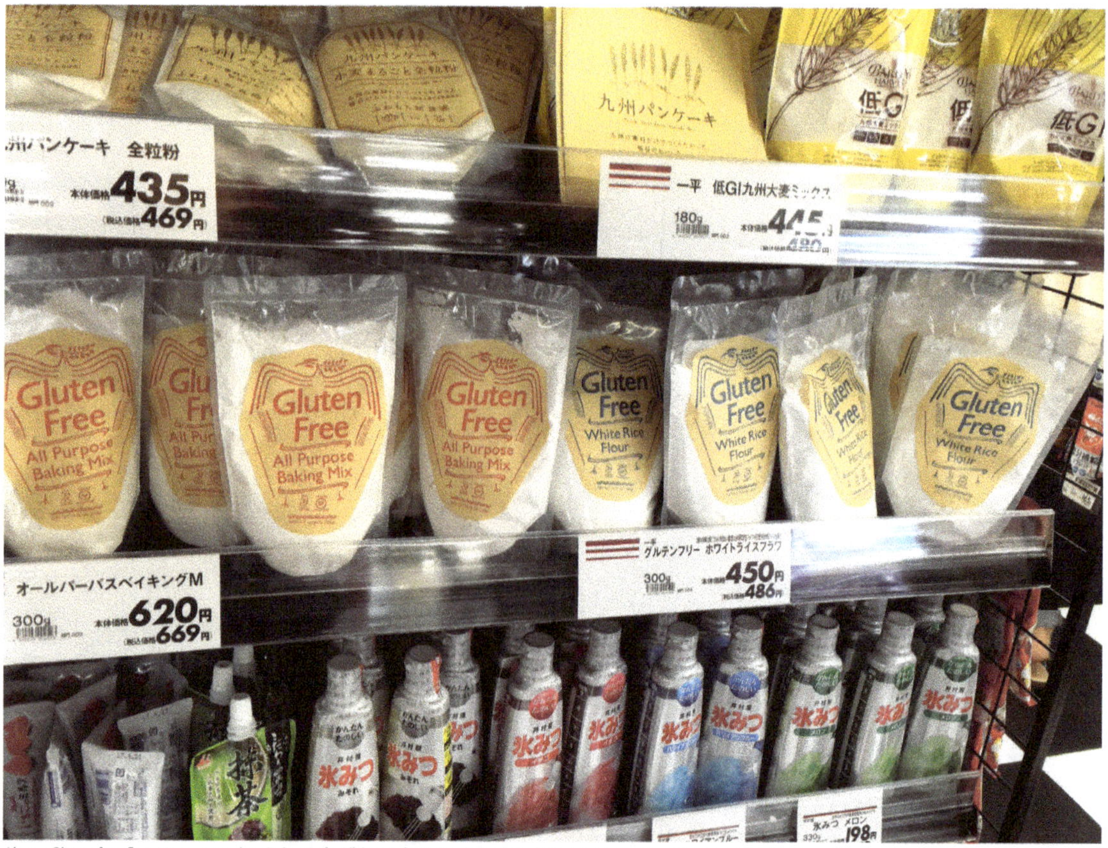

Above: Gluten-free flours in supermarket; Below Left: All Soyjoy bars are gluten-free; Below Right: Simple salt-grilled fish with rice, pickles and egg, from the supermarket

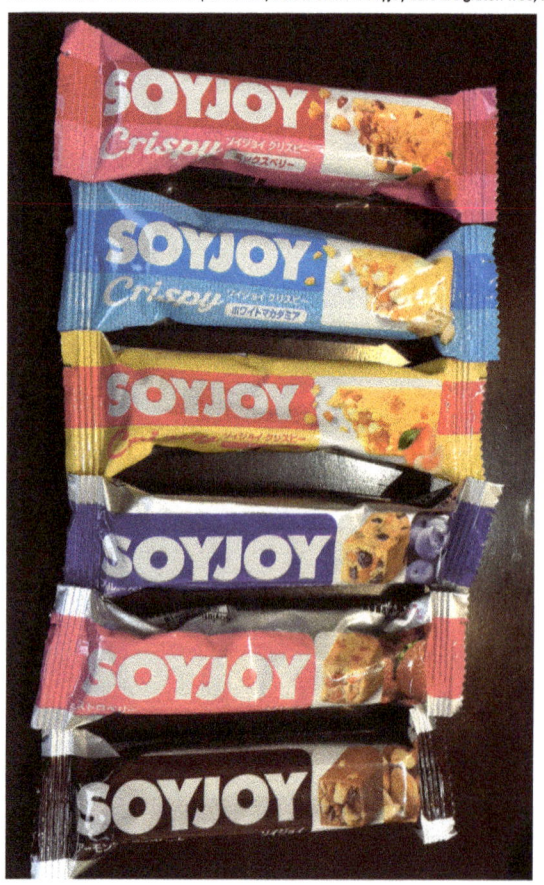

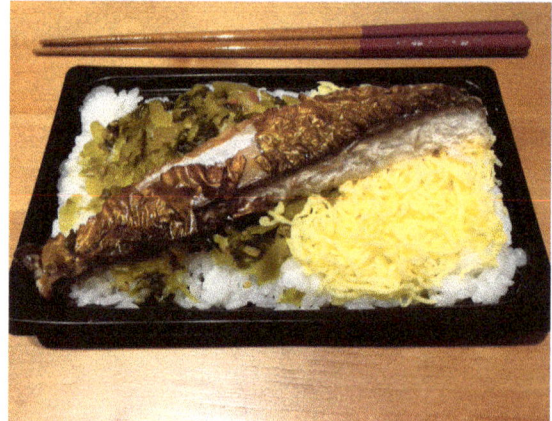

Below: Mochi (sweet rice balls) are often gluten-free

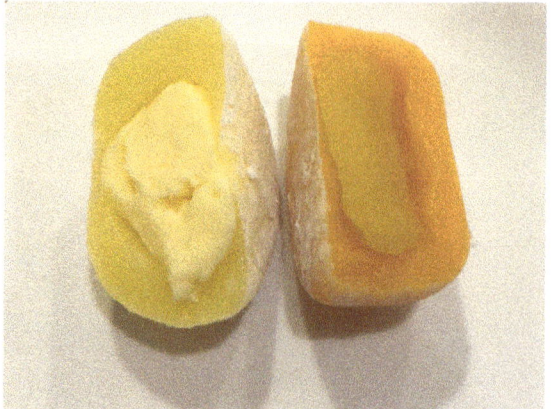

COELIAC DISEASE: Coeliac disease, genetics & gluten-free diet

Coeliac disease

Coeliac disease is a chronic inflammatory disease of the small intestine, a result of both environmental factors (allergy to dietary gluten from the cereals wheat, barley, rye and oats) and genetic factors. The villi that line the small intestine become atrophied and close up, reducing the normally large surface area through which essential nutrients are absorbed. In some people, coeliac disease is life-long, but it can also appear later in life. Symptoms of coeliac disease — including anaemia, osteoporosis, diarrhoea and weight loss — vary in type and severity from person to person. The only certain diagnosis is by small bowel biopsy, which allows an examination of the physical state of the intestinal villi.

Genetics

Coeliac disease is found in around one per cent of the world's population, but is predominantly a disease of the Western world. In ancient times, humans had a diet of meat, fruit and vegetables, until wild wheat and barley began to be cultivated in the Fertile Crescent of the Middle East. The spread of coeliac disease appears to have followed the migration routes of these early Middle Eastern wheat-eating Caucasian peoples. Today Australia and New Zealand have the highest rates of the disease, while China and Japan have amongst the lowest.

The genetic basis of coeliac disease involves several genes, the most important of which are on chromosome 6 — HLA-DQ2 and HLA-DQ8, which are involved in a 'restricted T-cell immune reaction' in the intestine. Populations of Japanese and Chinese ancestry, which have historically had little gluten in their diets, have a negligible frequency of HLA-DQ2 and therefore few diagnoses of coeliac disease — although the situation may be changing as more gluten-containing products are being consumed in Asia.

Gluten-free diet

On our first trip to Japan in 1991–1992 we loved the noodle dishes — ramen, soba, udon — and managed to get through a lot of other tempting gluten-packed foods such as tempura, cakes and bread. Not to mention enjoying Japan's well-known and delicious range of beers.

But when Bill was finally diagnosed with coeliac disease in his 50s, after four years of investigation by our GP, he would face considerable problems if we returned to Japan. Eating a gluten-free diet at home in Australia and in other western countries was fine because of the many alternative products that were available in the supermarkets, and, increasingly in restaurants. Whereas some Asian cuisines — such as Indian, Thai and Cambodian — are relatively 'safe' for coeliacs, the same can't be said for Japanese cuisine.

Although the Japanese diet is rice- rather than wheat-based, Japanese noodle dishes are widespread and very popular, but are practically all wheat-based. 100% buckwheat noodles (soba) are rare. Unfortunately the ubiquitous soy sauce used widely in most Japanese meals, in sauces and in snack foods like rice crackers — and even in dishes like omelettes, yakitori and grilled eel — is made using wheat. Supplies of gluten-free noodles and gluten-free soy sauce are not commonly available in Japan. And other common ingredients such as vinegar and miso, may not be gluten-free either, so both sushi and miso soup can be challenging for coeliacs who are at the extremity of sensitivity.

In Japan, several types of food can almost always be guaranteed to be gluten-free — such as sashimi, pickles, fresh fruit and vegetables, Macdonalds French fries, Soyjoy bars and grilled salted fish. Some others will be gluten-free as long as you specify 'no soy sauce' — such as donburi (rice bowls), tofu dishes, shabu-shabu (hot-pots) and salted yakitori. In the case of onigiri (savoury rice balls) and mochi (sweet rice balls), you'll need to look at the ingredients list.

Photo Page 9: Yatsuhoshi, a gluten-free Japanese confectionery made from glutinous rice flour, sugar and cinnamon and filled with red bean paste, sold mainly as an 'omiyage' or souvenirs in the Kyoto area

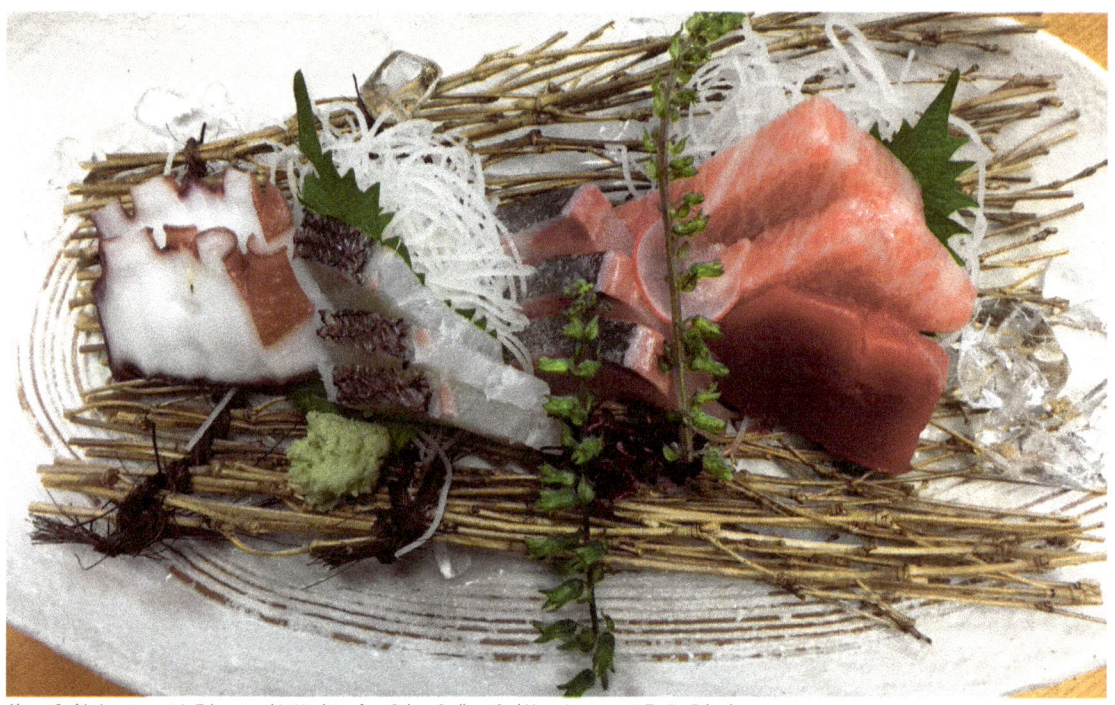
Above: Sashimi, restaurant in Tokyo — sashimi is gluten-free; Below: Scallops, Sushi Isogai restaurant, Tenjin, Fukuoka

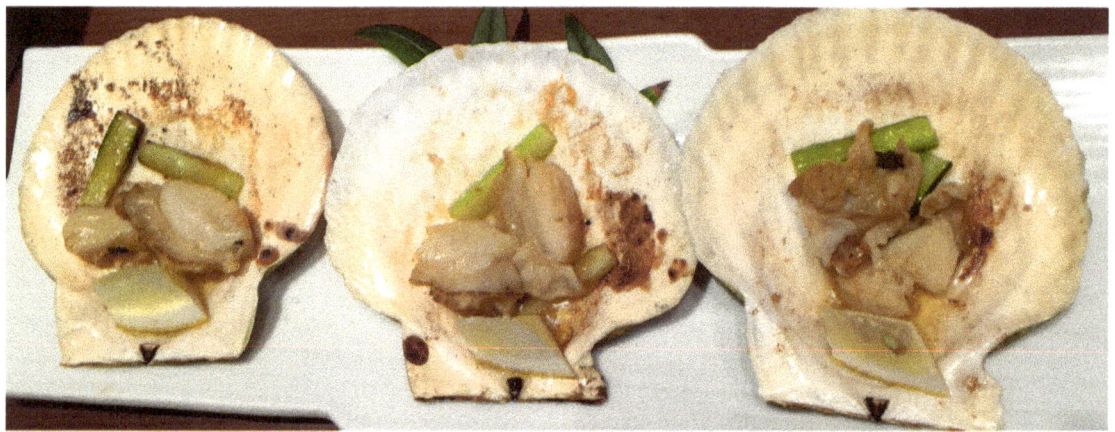
Below Left: Gluten-free soy sauce bought at large department store in Tokyo; Below Right: Kaldi Coffee Farms sell a range of foreign and gluten-free groceries

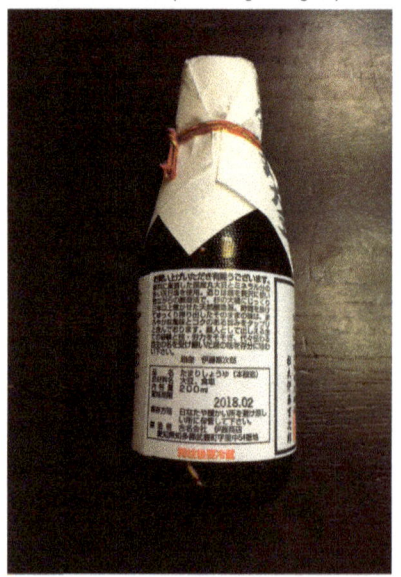
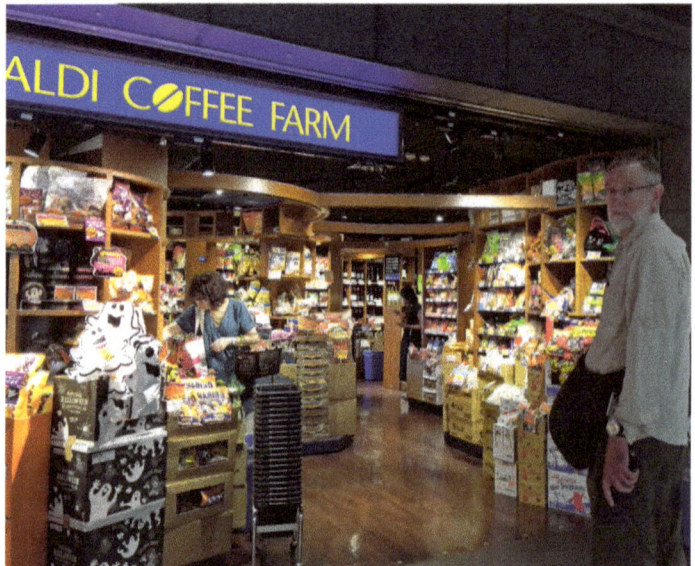

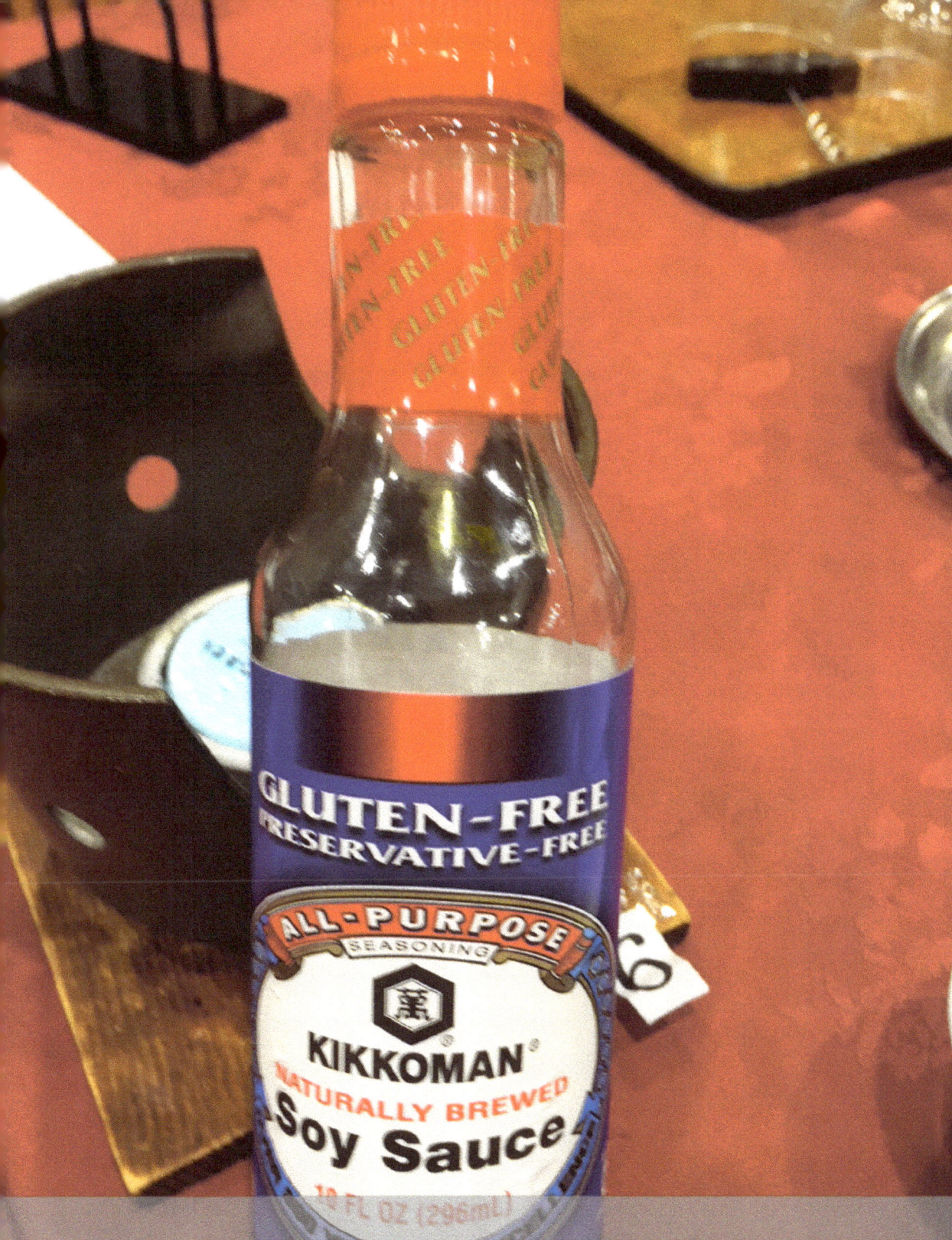

Planning your trip
Where to go, where to stay & what to do

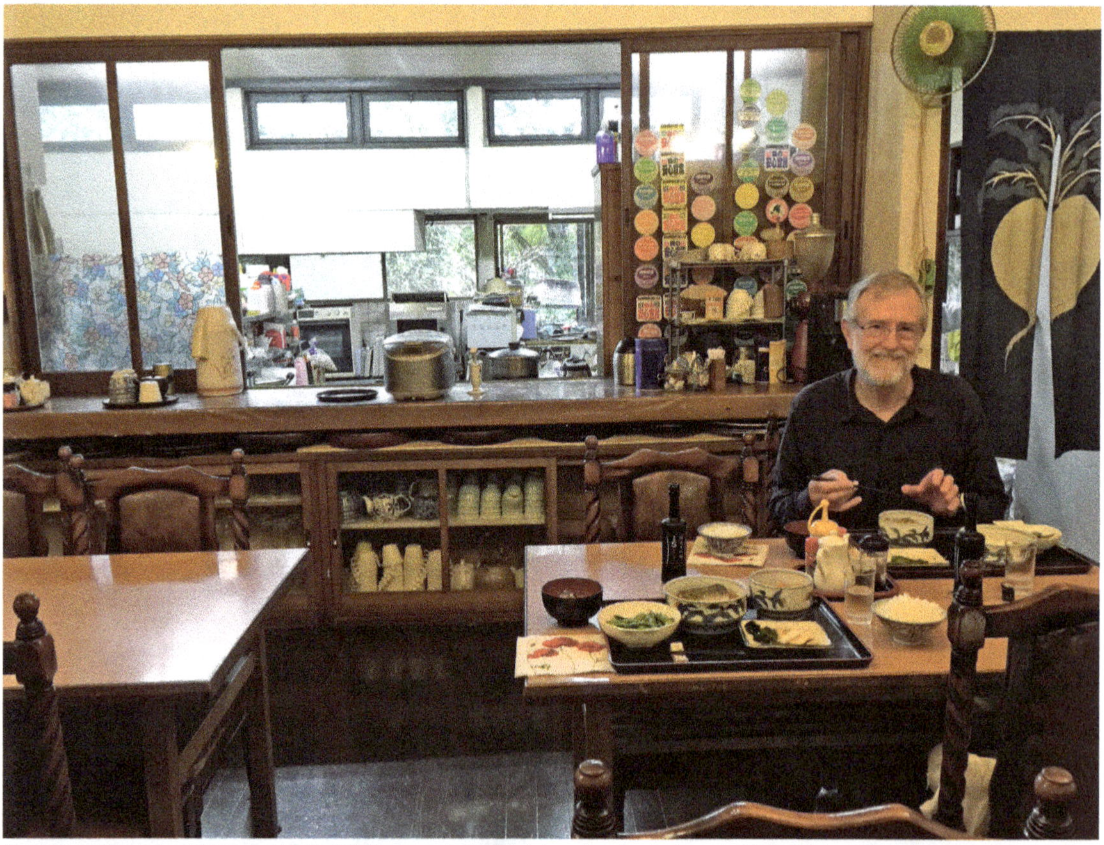

Above: Dinner, Nikko Suginamiki Youth Hostel; Below Left: Miso soup with Hokkaido baby scallops, Pension Arumeria, Wakkanai; Below Right: Barbecue restaurant, Tsuruoka

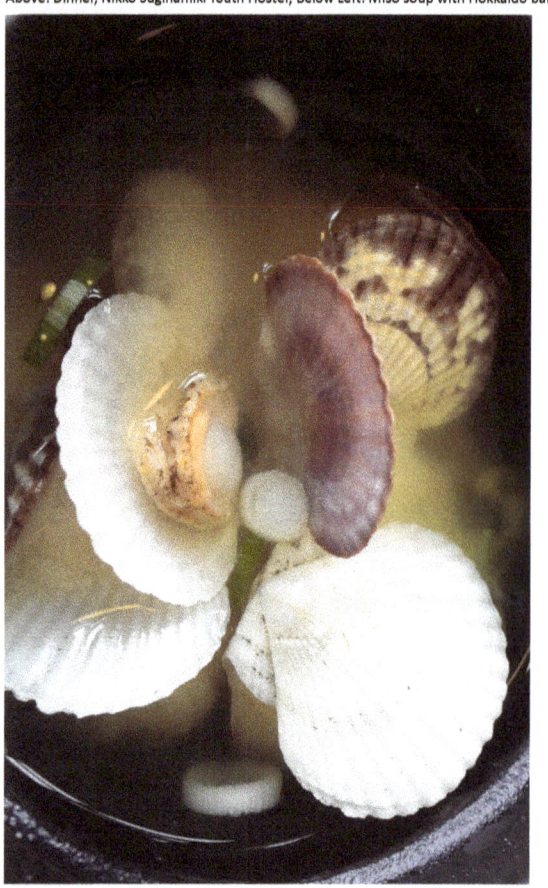
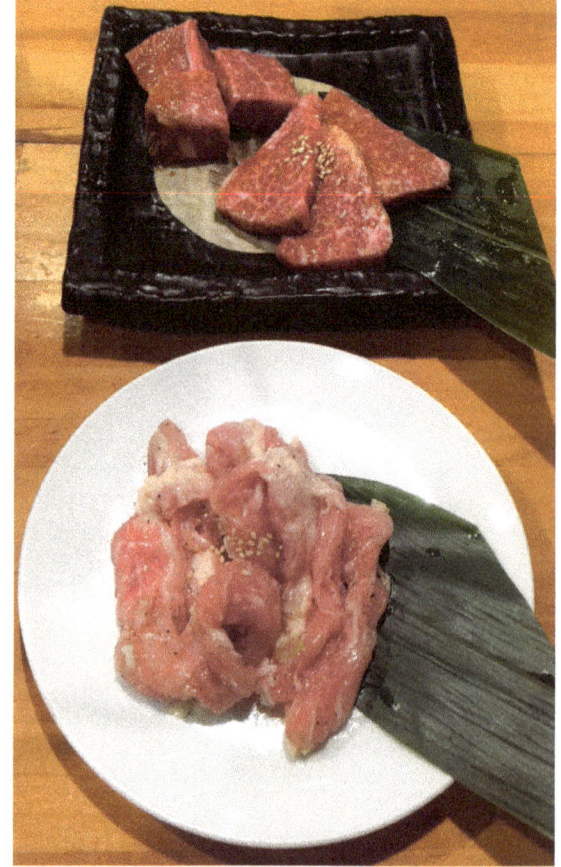

PLANNING YOUR TRIP: Where to go, where to stay & what to do

Where to go

Planning where to go in Japan depends on your particular interests and what season(s) you will be travelling. Being keen walkers, we planned our year around two long-distance walks, booked with a tour company that had bilingual tour guides who would be able to help organise our special dietary requirements.

Our itinerary was also dictated by the weather. Having been to Japan in the middle of winter on our first visit, we decided to avoid the cold weather. We started our trip at a language school in Fukuoka in September and October so that we would be largely indoors during the worst of the typhoon season. After language school we did our autumn walk starting from Osaka, before heading back south and spending the winter in subtropical Okinawa, then worked our way up to central Honshu via Shikoku for the second walk starting in Kyoto. Two months in the Kyoto-Tokyo area is barely enough, so make sure to factor in as much time as possible there! After Tokyo we continued, in the spring, to make our way north to spend the summer months in Hokkaido, away from the hot humid conditions in central and southern Japan.

We travelled right through Japan, from the Yaeyama Islands in the south to Rebun Island in the north — so you might get some ideas from our other book *Budget Travel in Japan*.

Where to stay

Planning accommodation will depend on your preferences and budget. But wherever you stay, if you want to book meals, you'll find most places will cater for a gluten-free diet if you explain the requirements. If you don't know any Japanese try using Google Translate or a restaurant card (see Introduction).

With a whole year in Japan, we had to economise with accommodation. Our school arranged for us to rent a tiny apartment for our first two months in Fukuoka. After that we used a mix of Airbnbs, hotels, hostels, Youth Hostels and 'ryokans' (traditional inns). The ryokan accommodation provided on our walks was excellent, while the Airbnbs were not only good value but allowed us to live like the locals and often mingle with hosts or neighbours. The hostel chain we used was 'K's House', a series of clean, efficiently run, friendly places that were both economical and well located in the main tourist centres. Relatively cheap hotels were easy to come by and useful when we needed to stay close to a station. Most provided a buffet breakfast with plenty of gluten-free options (avoid the ones offering only continental breakfasts!). Youth Hostels were great too. Often located out of town, most had spacious private rooms available (often with own bathroom), and the hosts were friendly and would provide breakfasts and dinners if you booked early enough.

What to do

While some of our best experiences were planned in advance, many were unplanned chance encounters or snap decisions based on recommendations from people we met along the way, from information counters, or from reading *Lonely Planet* as we journeyed around. In Japan, it's fair to say that tourists should expect the unexpected, and that even the most out-of-the-way or unlikely places will have some unique experience to offer. In a way, this makes planning easy. All you have to do is decide on the main places you want to visit, and go to other places along the way.

What gluten-free supplies to pack before you leave your home country

Gluten-free cooking ingredients such as flour and soy sauce are hard to find in Japan, so it's a good idea to pack a few supplementary supplies. One or two bottles of carefully packed soy sauce, a jar of GF vegemite and a packet of flour will be handy, especially if you are likely to be cooking. You can take packaged bread in your luggage if there's room. However, why not throw yourself in at the deep end and with our advice, go and find some local meals that are gluten-free!

Photo Page 13: Soy sauce bought in Australia and taken in our luggage

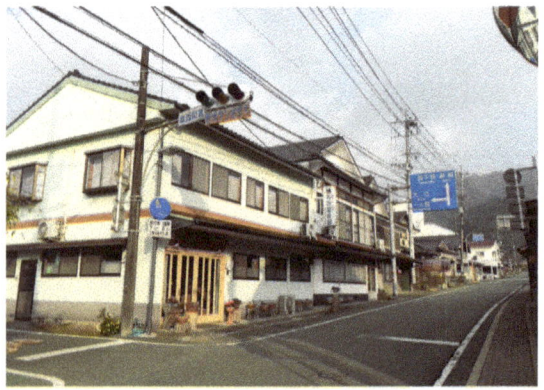

Above: Youth Hostel Murataya Ryokan, Takamori

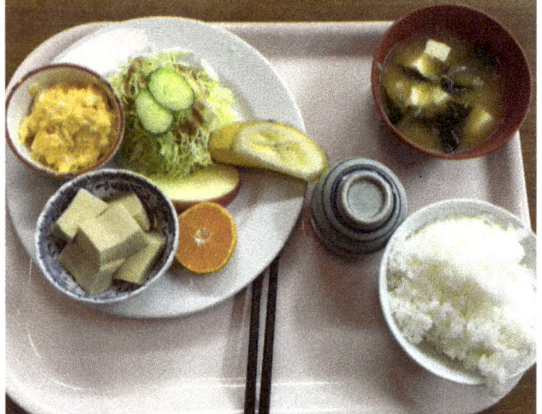

Above: Breakfast at Youth Hostel, Kurashiki

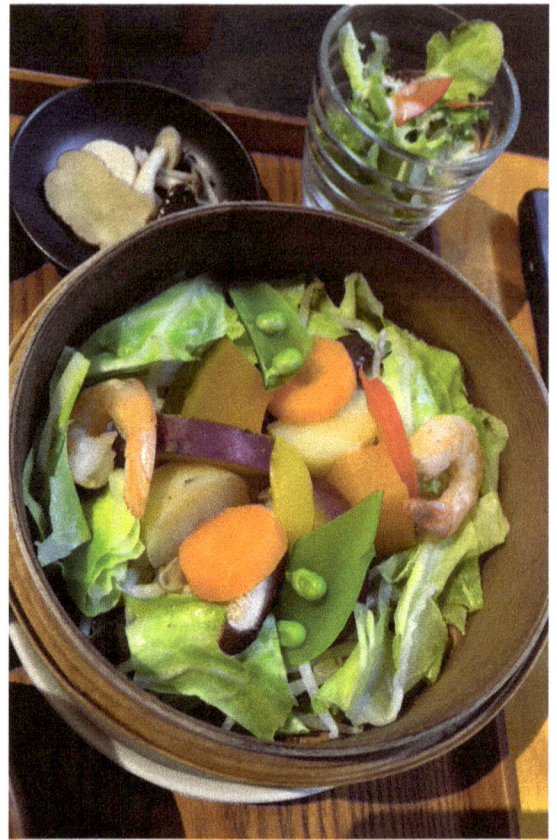

Above & Below: Meal and dining room at That Sounds Good Jazz Pension, Tazawako

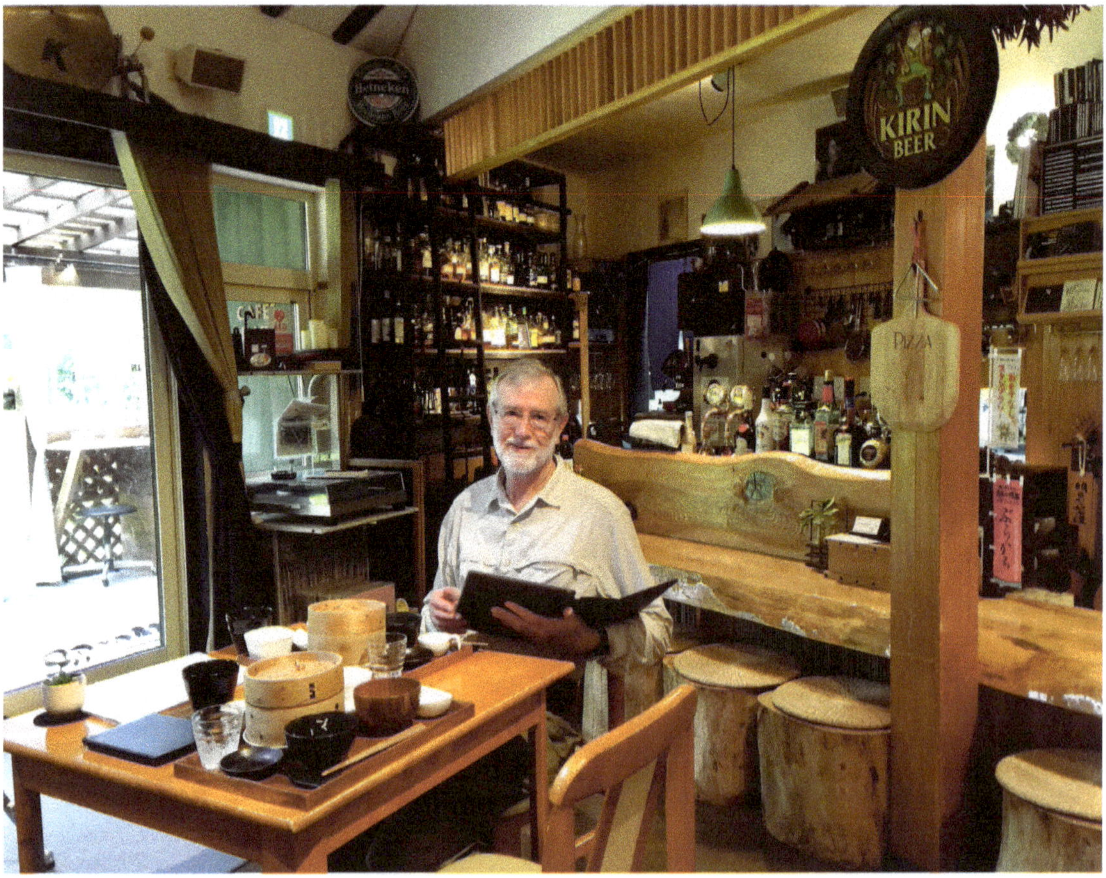

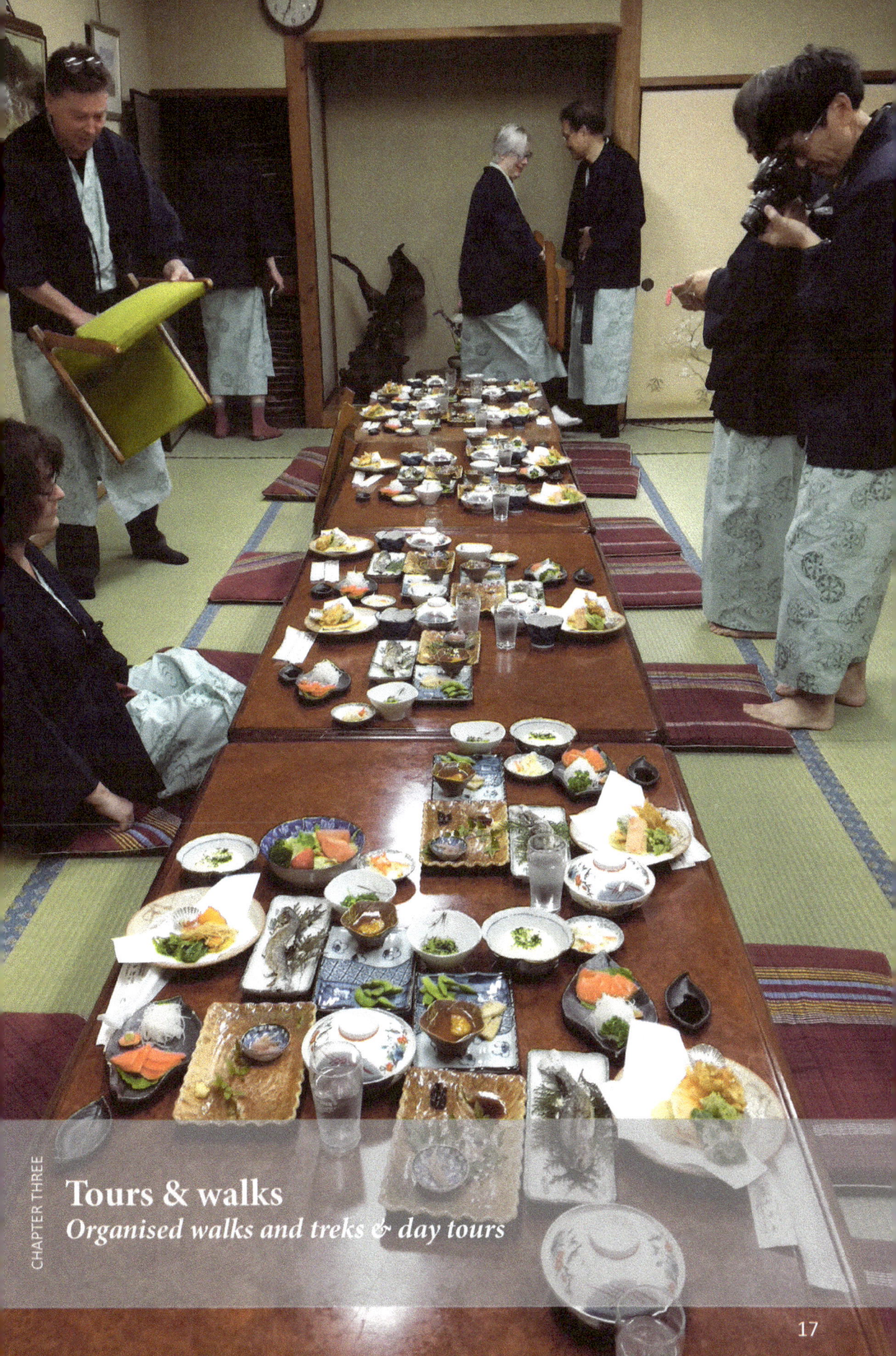

Tours & walks
Organised walks and treks & day tours

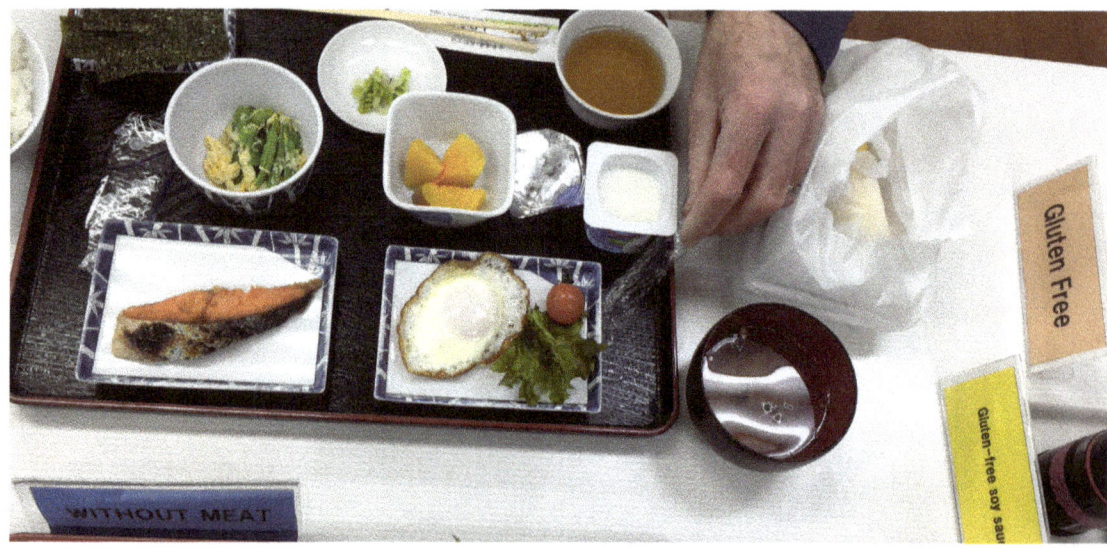
Above: Gluten-free breakfast at Koguchi, on the Kumano-Kodo walk, with labelled gluten-free soy sauce

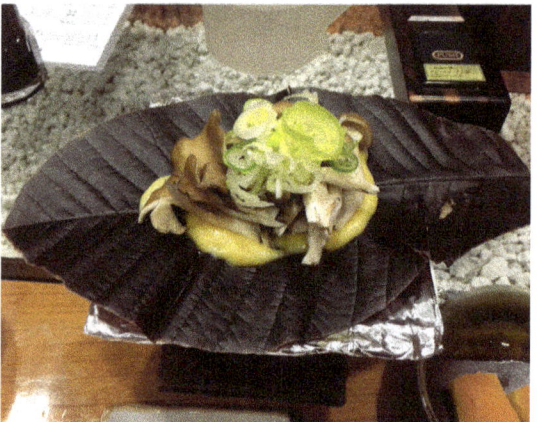
Above: Miso vegetables on magnolia leaf, Nakasendo Way walk

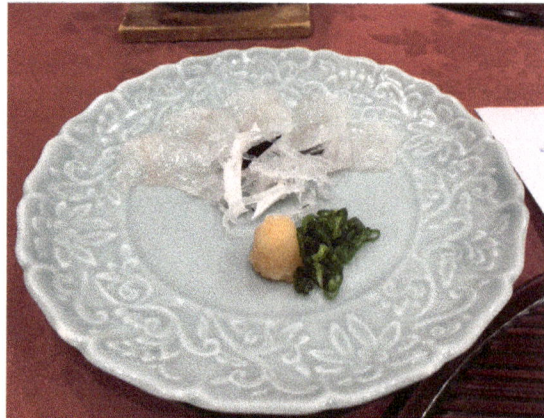
Above: Blowfish sashimi; Below: Picnic snacks from village shop, Nakasendo Way

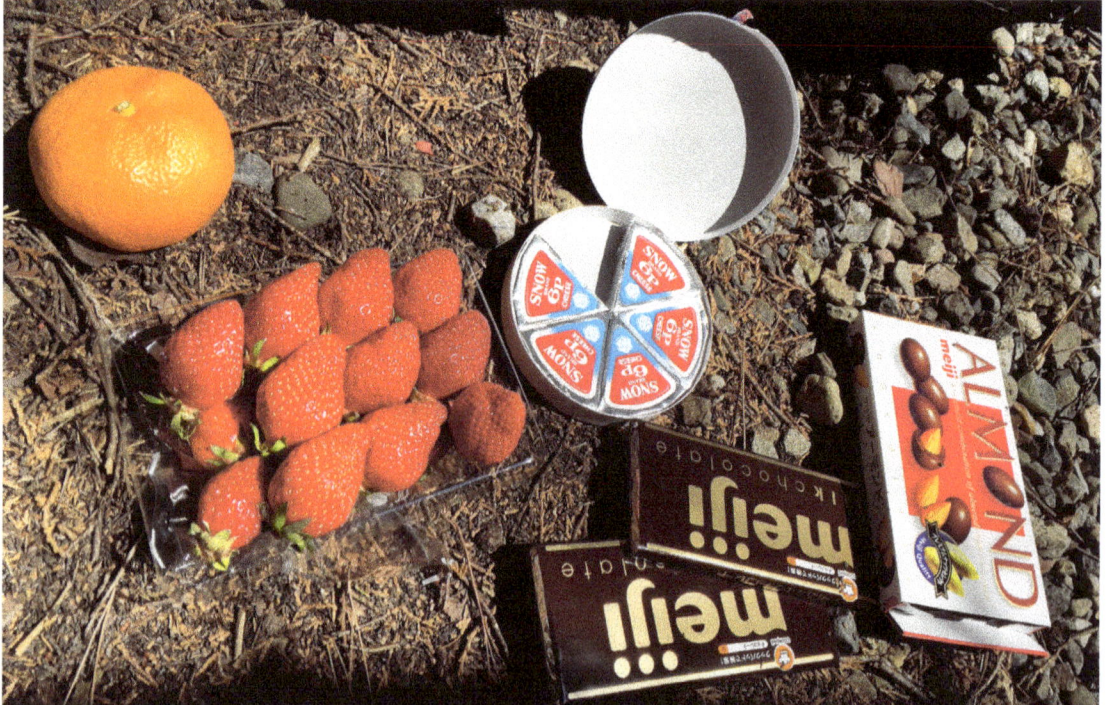

TOURS & WALKS: Communicating dietary requirements

Organised walks and treks

In order to avoid dietary problems on our two walks (treks of nine and eleven days), we booked with a tour company. The main benefit of booking with a tour company — rather than organising a walk yourself — is that the company provides one or two guides who speak your own language in addition to Japanese. Our guides not only had a good knowledge of the history, culture and landscape but they were able to organise meals around our dietary requirements and deal with any problems that arose.

We booked both our walks in advance with a tour company before leaving Australia. After filling out the 'dietary requirements' section of the booking form for gluten-free meals, we were subsequently informed that although the company couldn't guarantee to provide vegetarian, vegan, kosher, or other specific meals, they would endeavour to cater, wherever possible, to individual needs.

They did this remarkably well. We were advised at the tour briefing to bring our own gluten-free snacks but that our breakfasts and dinners would be catered for as best as possible. Along the way, our accommodations did indeed provide sumptuous evening meals and delicious breakfasts. There was usually a specially prepared gluten-free meal, with an accompanying label. Although the regular meals were generous and comprised many different dishes, non-gluten-free soy sauce was such a common ingredient that if we hadn't taken our own bottle of gluten-free soy sauce Bill's choices would have been quite limited. Our guides helped if there were any problems and they also understood why we sometimes chose to eat lunch at different restaurants from the rest of the group!

The only real problems we encountered were with lunches — for example if there was a small restaurant that only served noodle dishes, or if we had to buy picnic lunch ingredients from a small grocery store in the countryside. In the case of the former, a bowl of rice, and with the latter, fruit and cheese, had to suffice. We soon learnt to keep a supply of Soyjoy bars and rice crackers (see Chapter 10) in our day packs. These are available at convenience stores or supermarkets.

Day tours

During our time in Japan we did several bus day tours, organised either online or at an office at the city's main bus station. They can be especially useful if you don't have a hire car, as each tour usually goes to several different places of interest that may be far apart and not easily reached by public transport on the same day. Bus tours tend to be lengthy, but with a knowledgeable guide, comfy seats and plenty of comfort stops, they are a good way to see the sights economically.

Bus tours have comfort stops at roadhouses where there is a wide variety of food and drinks for sale. However, it's advisable to take your own snacks, just in case! The stopping places usually feature a plethora of 'omiyage' (souvenirs), many of which are edible and some of which are gluten-free. You just might not have time to use Google Translate on the ingredients of the packaging before it's time to re-board the bus, so simply look for the characters for wheat, barley, rye and oats (keep photos of them on your phone). If the bus tour includes lunch, it is likely to be a buffet with plenty of choices. If in doubt, ask your tour guide to quiz the staff. The lunch venue will be given in the itinerary and is most likely to be a hotel or large restaurant, although it could be a sushi place.

> **What gluten-free supplies to carry with you on walks or bus trips**
>
> We had a bag of supplies that was transported with our luggage on the organised walks, but wherever we were in Japan we had snacks in our day packs. The best gluten-free snacks are Soyjoy bars (which come in a dozen or so flavours) and rice crackers are also handy. Rice crackers are branded with Japanese characters, so you'll have to check that the wheat character isn't amongst the ingredients — or ask — then photograph the packet so you can find them again next time.

Photo Page 17: Dinner at Shinchaya on Nakasendo Way walk

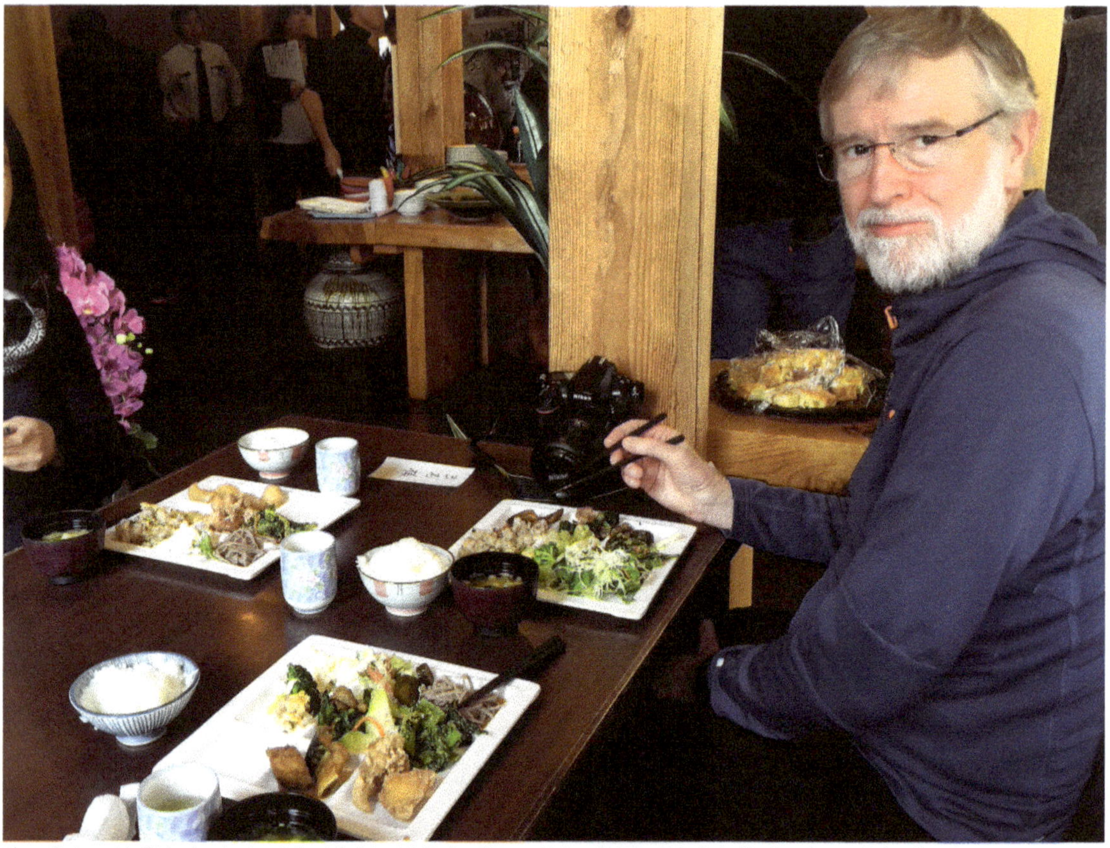

Above: Restaurant buffet lunch on bus tour; Below Left: Hot-pot, Sekigahara, Kumano-Kodo walk; Below Right: Packed lunch on Kumano-Kodo walk

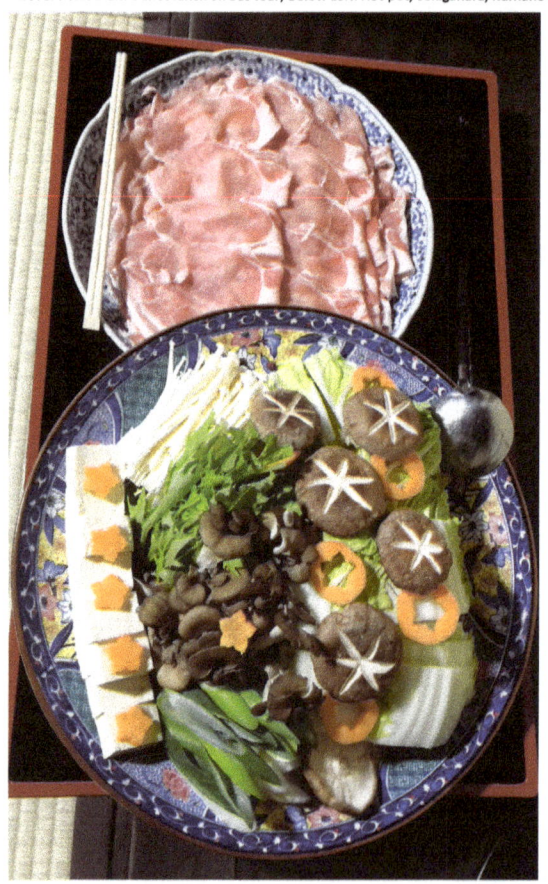
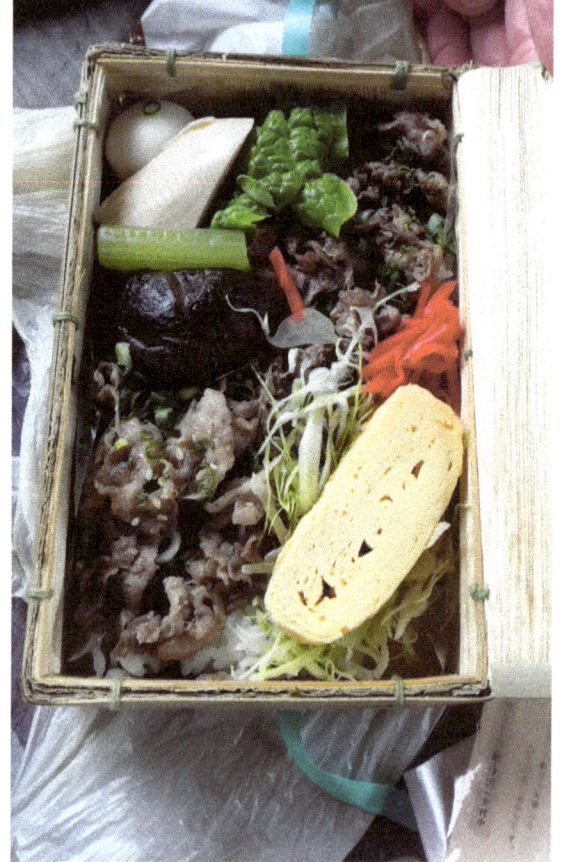

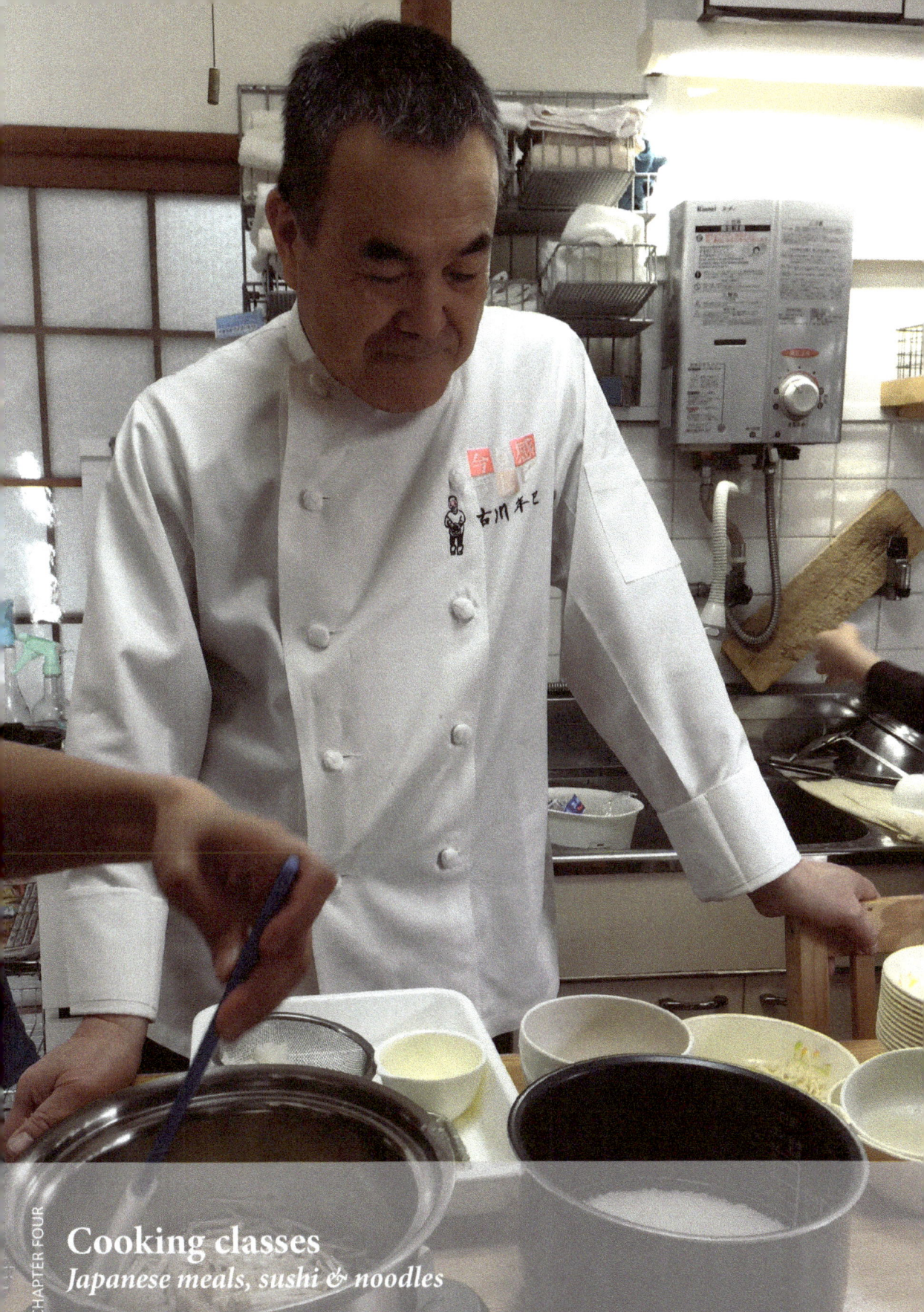

CHAPTER FOUR

Cooking classes
Japanese meals, sushi & noodles

21

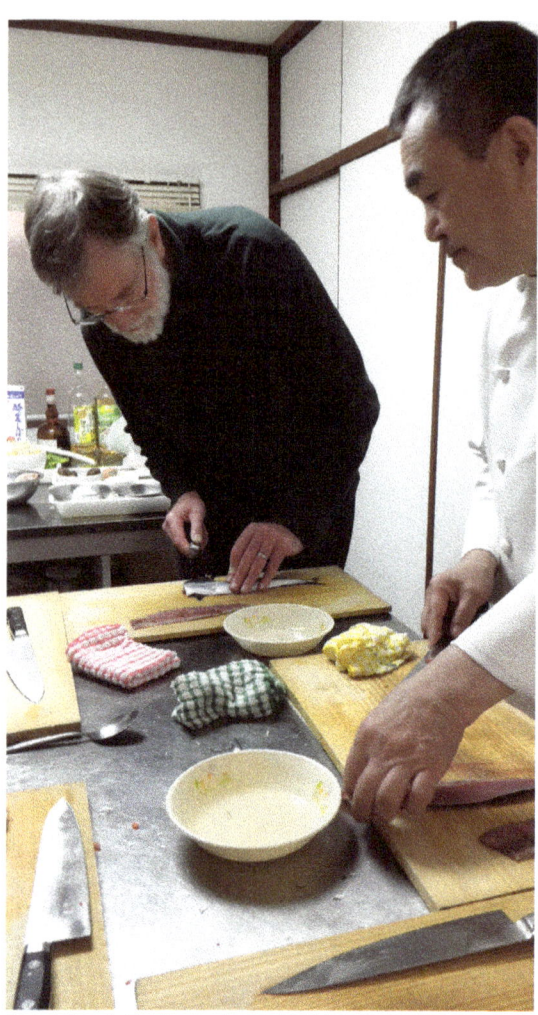

Above & Right: Cooking class, Furukawa Cooking School, Ohashi

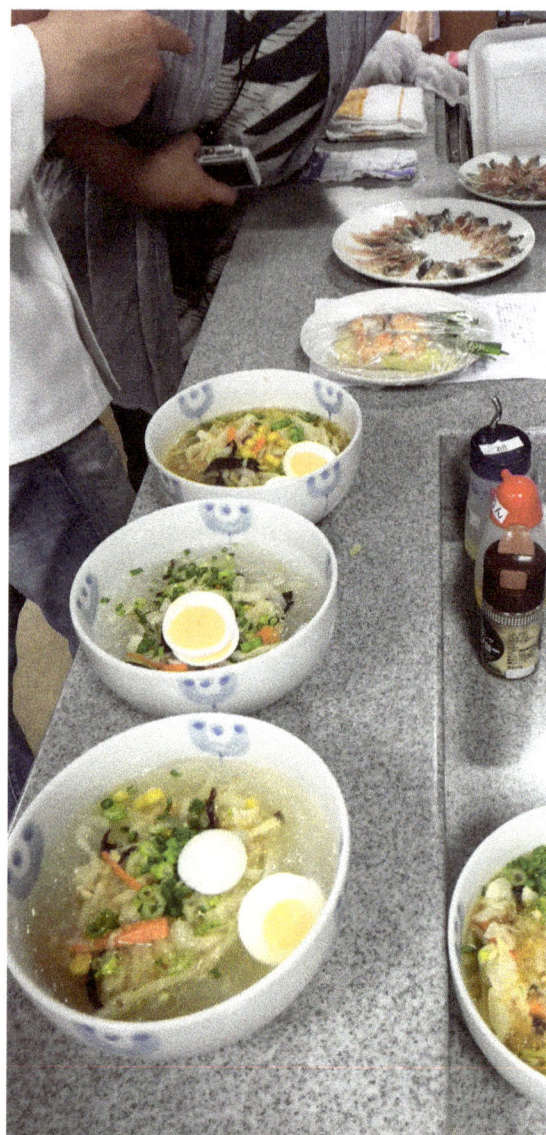

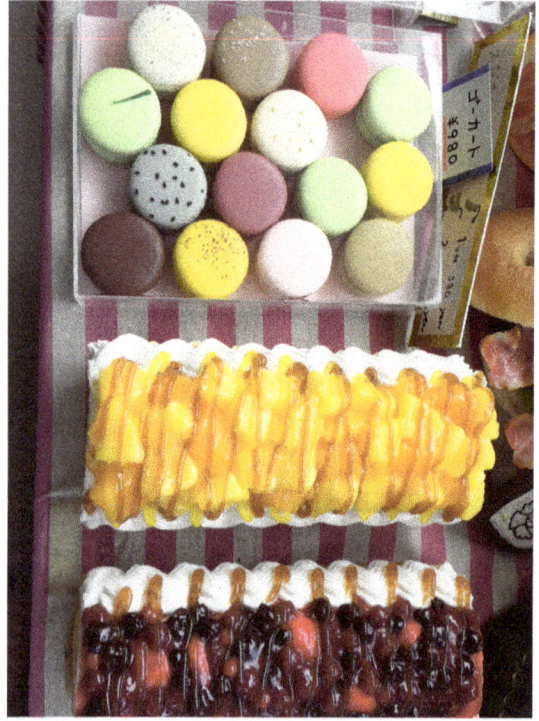

Left: Fake food Workshop Riki; Below: Gluten-free rice vinegar used in sushi class

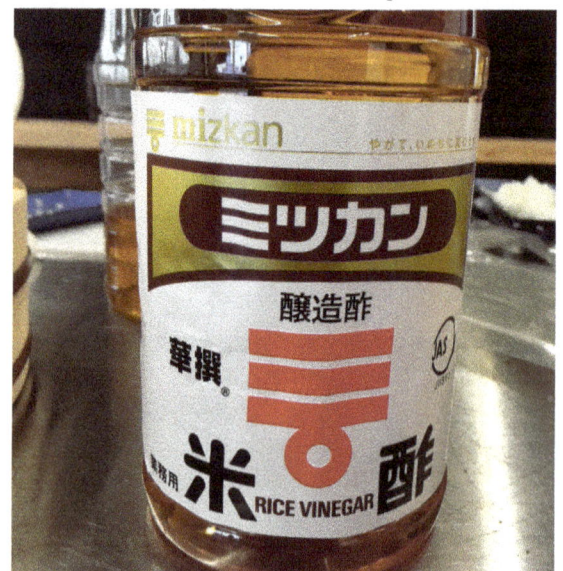

COOKING CLASSES: Japanese meals, sushi and noodles

Cooking a Japanese meal

While it's fun and interesting to learn some Japanese cooking during your stay in Japan, it can understandably be hard to muster any enthusiasm if you're coeliac and unlikely to be able to eat the food you are learning to cook.

But don't be put off! We found that people go out of their way to accommodate dietary preferences as long as you explain them clearly. If soy sauce is a problem ingredient, take your own — we did this for a rice cracker-making class. Cooking classes give you the opportunity to see at first hand what ingredients go into local dishes and to closely examine the labels along the way. If all else fails, try your hand at making fake food — which no-one can eat!

We attended two very enjoyable cooking classes in Fukuoka, organised by our language school and run by teacher Furukawa-san, a former TV cooking show celebrity who is an entertaining cook and a good teacher. Our first class was held in a large teaching kitchen that accommodated several groups, including our school group and a group of doctors. A later class, however, was held in an apartment with a cosy home-like atmosphere more suited to a small group.

We cooked slightly different meals each time, but on both occasions Furukawa-san took note of everyone's food allergies and preferences and varied the menus or ingredients accordingly. For example, for coeliacs he cooked a separate hotpot, using vermicelli and gluten-free soy sauce. Other ingredients — fish, vegetables, rice, rice vinegar — were gluten-free, or in the case of dumplings, simply omitted.

The dishes we prepared were typical of local Fukuoka cuisine — sashimi, rice paper rolls, soup, and noodle hot-pot with meat and dumplings. In one class we prepared the fish carpacchio style, and in the other we seared the fish using a kitchen blow torch. The highlights were learning how to cut a fish into wafer-thin slices for sashimi — not an easy job, but we managed to obtain a reasonably professional result — and enjoying the group meal at the end of the class.

Making sushi

A sushi-making class is a real eye-opener. It takes many years to become an accomplished sushi chef, and we soon found out why! It's not nearly as easy as it looks. Not only to make the sushi, but also to learn how to plate the pieces so they are eaten in the correct order, at the correct orientation, and with the correct garnishes. Of course, there's quite a bit of history and cultural background behind every step in the process that sushi chefs also have to absorb in their training.

Our class was held at Suito in Fukuoka, under the direction of a sushi chef. During the class we learnt the correct way to prepare sushi rice and noted that all ingredients the chef used were gluten-free and of high quality. The seafood was very fresh but was, surprisingly, handled over and over through a series of set manoeuvres when attaching the fish/prawn/etc. to the rice ball base. An expert would probably have a lighter touch than us, and we will have to put in a bit of practice if we want to impress anyone!

Making noodles

Ramen noodles are an important part of the cuisine of Fukuoka. We decided to do the ramen (noodles) and gyoza (pork dumplings) class at Child Kitchen because friends assured us the class would be fun even if we didn't get to eat the results. The class was very enjoyable, with some unexpected techniques (such as flattening the dough by stomping on it with your feet). It was satisfying to make the ramen and gyoza from scratch and useful to see what ingredients were used.

Soba (buckwheat) noodles are more typical of the mountainous areas of Japan and we had a lesson on making them at the Tonkururen Togakushi Soba Museum near Nagano. Throughout Japan, soba noodles usually contain a percentage of wheat flour and so are not suitable for coeliacs. The best advice is to avoid soba, though occasionally you can find 100% buckwheat soba in specialty supermarkets and some restaurants (see Chapter 21). Nevertheless, the class was well run, fun and interesting — and we can now try to make soba at home using 100% buckwheat flour.

23

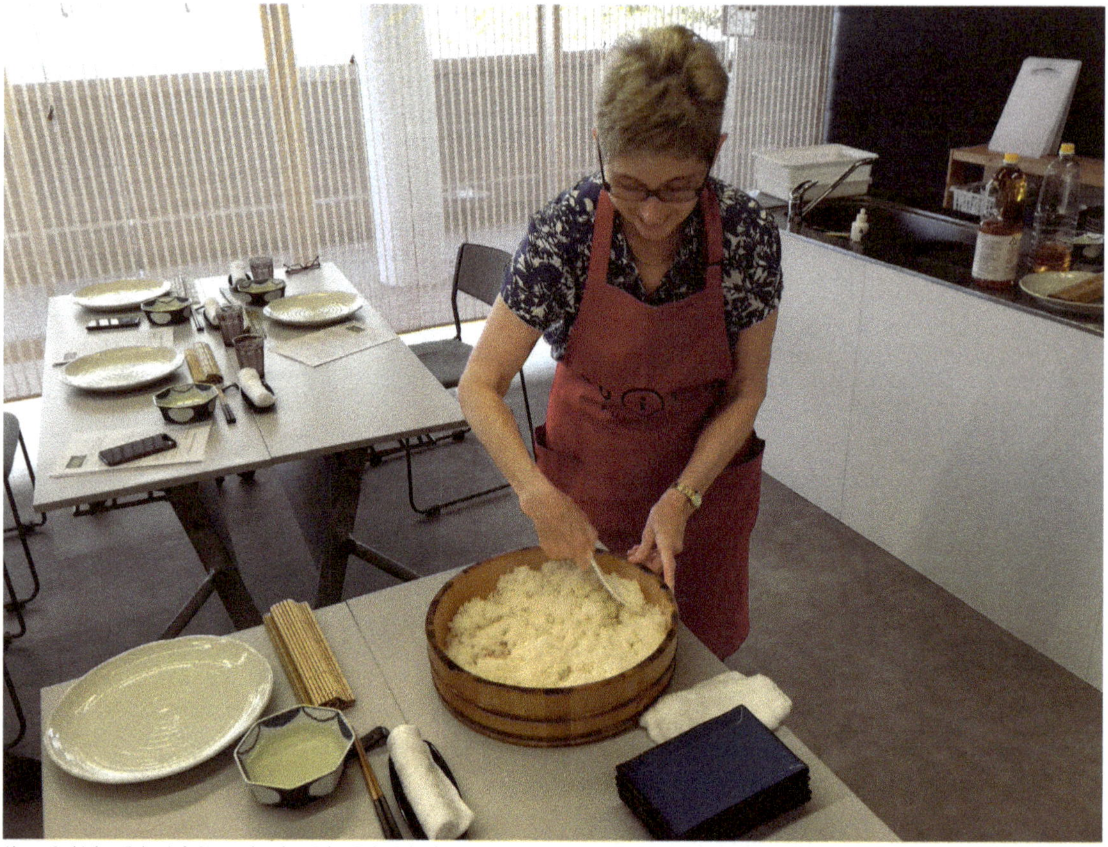

Above: Sushi class; Below Left: Rice cracker class; Below Right: Soba class

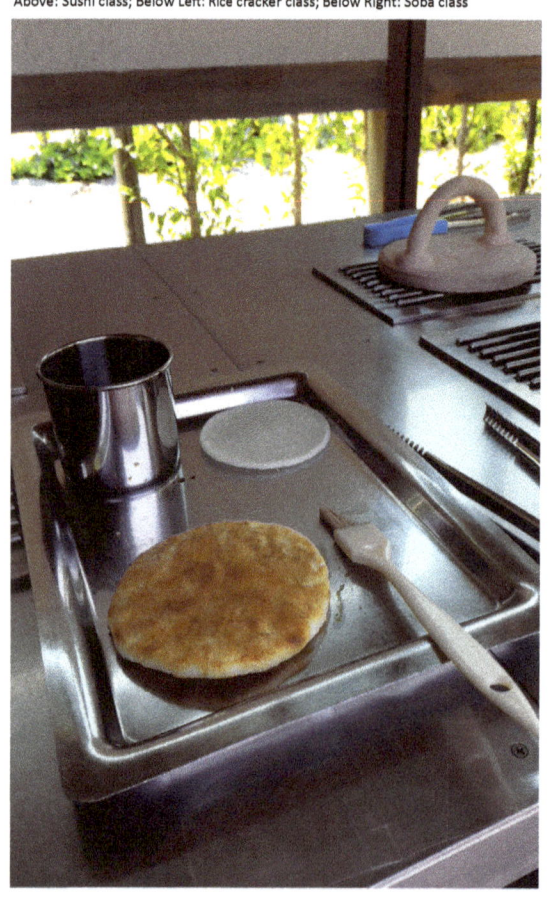
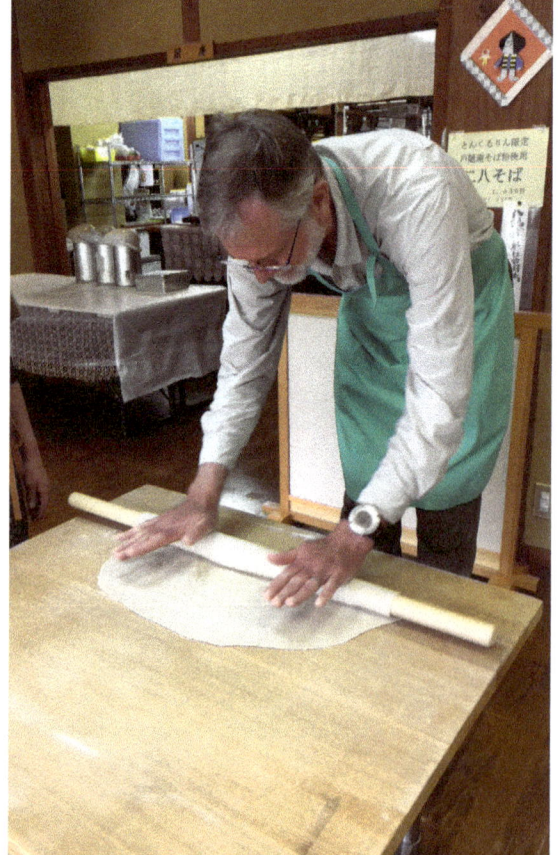

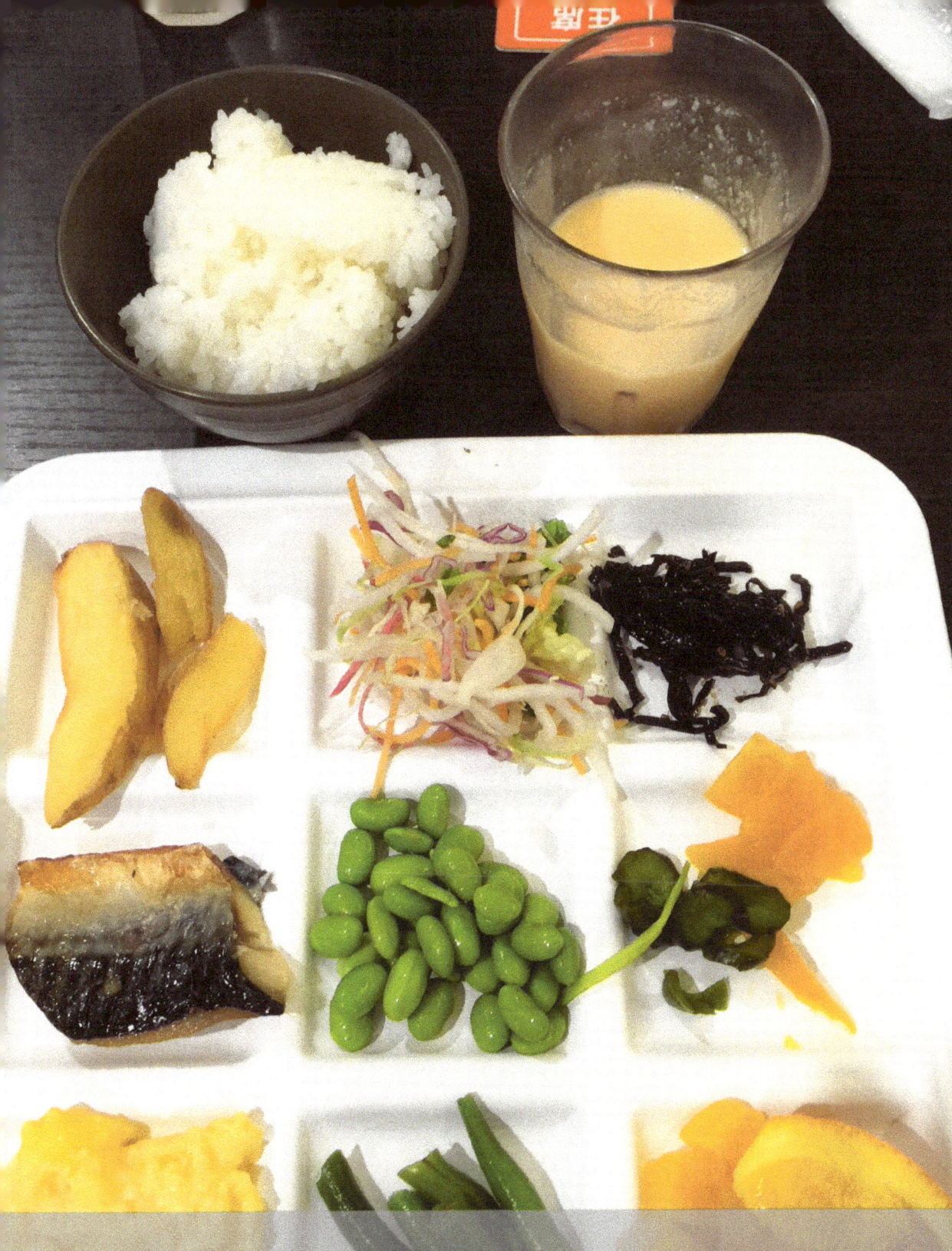

CHAPTER FIVE
Hotels
Breakfasts, lunches and dinners & eating in

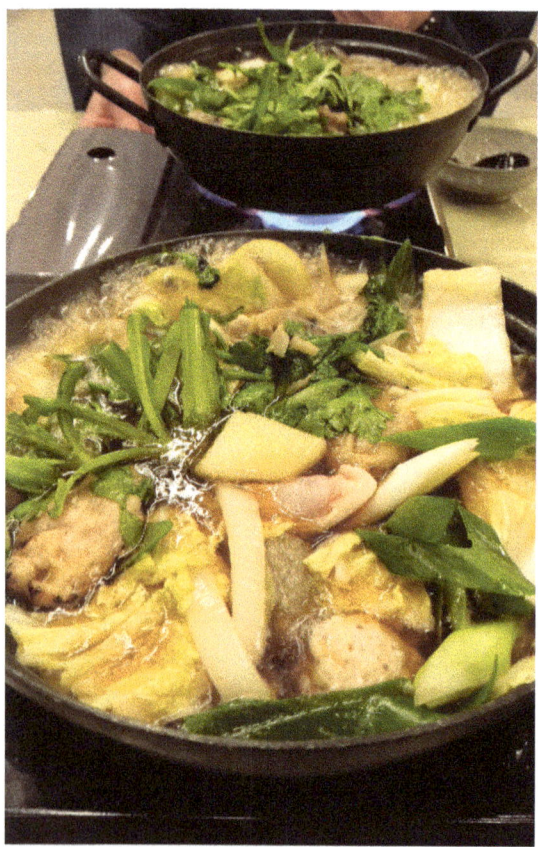

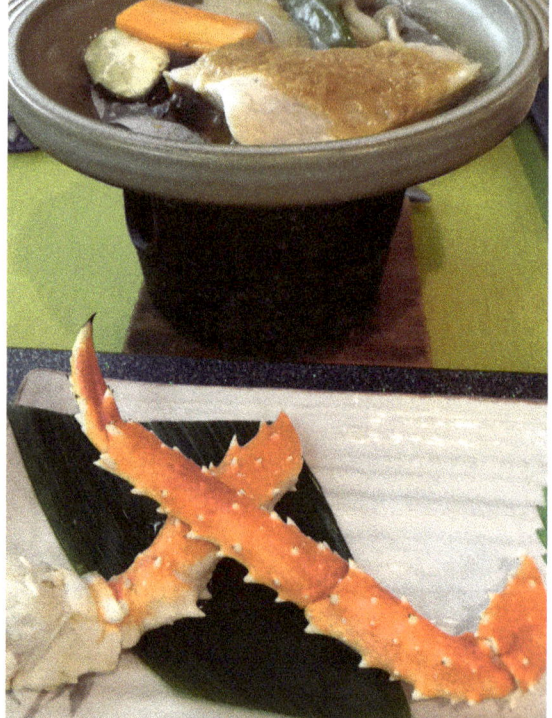

Above: Hot-pot dinner in Tsuwano; Below: Gluten-free dinner menu Benesse House

Above: Touakarino Yado Rausu Daiichi Hotel, Rausu; Below: Supermarket takeaways

KAISEKI ZEN -禅-

November 霜月

Appetizer
Assorted seasonal appetizer

Cup
Chawan-mushi cup egg custard

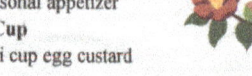

Sashimi
Thin-sliced Konnyaku / Soy milk skin

Fried dish
Fried pumpkin bun glazed with Yoshino-Kudzu sauce

Grilled dish
Grilled eggplant with miso

Steamed dish
Steamed vegetables

Additional dish
Boiled Tofu

Rice
Rice, miso soup and pickles

Fruit
Raspberry and mango sherbets

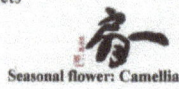

Seasonal flower: Camellia

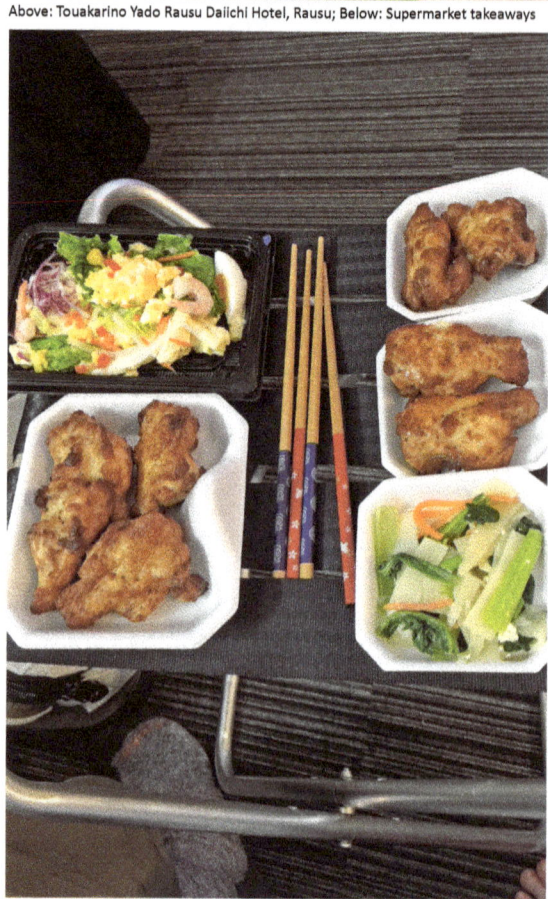

HOTELS: Breakfasts, lunches and dinners & eating in

Breakfasts

Most of the hotels we stayed at in Japan were two- or three- star business hotels, which were reasonably priced and usually near railway stations, chosen to suit late arrivals or early departures, without having to carry bags very long distances. Occasionally we stayed at more luxurious hotels with something special to offer or if there was little other alternative.

Booking hotels online at the last minute isn't usually a problem, although accommodation can be hard to find if there's a festival on or if it's peak tourist time — such as during cherry blossom viewing ('hanami'), Golden Week, or around New Year. When making a booking you'll usually have the option of paying ahead for breakfast to be included. Do it, the breakfasts are great value! By and large the breakfasts are buffet style with a mix of Western and Asian foods. The buffets are excellent because they feature many gluten-free choices and the staff are always willing to explain what the dishes are and what goes into them, if you ask. Some of the foods on offer at hotel buffet breakfasts include juices, fish, eggs, rice, fruit, pickles, salads, yoghurt and miso soup. They also feature the usual breads and cereals unsuitable for coeliacs.

At a few of the hotels we came across, there was either one or a choice of several set breakfast trays, the components of which were mostly suitable for coeliacs. Our breakfast at the Kinoe Sou in Kamoenai in Hokkaido was especially memorable. If you're travelling with a partner or friend who doesn't have to stick to a gluten-free diet, a certain amount of swapping between trays always helps! Infrequently you'll find hotels that offer only a continental breakfast that features wheat-packed breads and cereals — so we avoided those particular places.

Lunches and dinners

Few of the business hotels we stayed at had lunches or dinners available — but in the main there were heaps of restaurants in the near vicinity. Hotels in more isolated locations in the countryside often had restaurants with excellent dinners. Again, it's advisable to enquire about the menu beforehand at these restaurants as the staff are usually very helpful and will oblige with gluten-free options. Unless the restaurant is a pizza/pasta place. Occasionally when we hadn't booked for dinner at the hotel in advance, we found it was too late to do so once we arrived. In those cases the hotel staff would usually recommend somewhere nearby to eat.

We enjoyed some amazingly good dinners at slightly more expensive hotels located out of town with no nearby restaurants. Examples included the Shuho Royal Hotel Shuhokan at Mine, and the Tsuwano Hotel (an excellent hot-pot), both in Honshu, and the Touakarino Yado Rausu Daiichi Hotel in Hokkaido.

Our most exquisite hotel meals were at Benesse House, in Naoshima — one of the Art Islands in the Inland Sea off Shikoku. The hotel was recommended by friends because of its many site-specific artworks that can only be viewed by overnighting guests, and free entry to Benesse House Museum was included. Benesse House was the most expensive hotel we stayed at and we had to book well in advance for accommodation and meals, for which we requested gluten-free for one guest. The breakfasts were delicious buffets in a restaurant overlooking the Inland Sea. For dinner we had our own multi-course menus in the Museum Restaurant Issen, which featured some Andy Warhol artworks.

Eating in

While hotels don't usually provide cooking facilities in your room, they will have an electric jug for boiling water, as well as a small fridge. If there isn't a hotel restaurant or any nearby place for dinner, or if you're simply feeling lazy or can't afford to dine out every night, most hotels don't mind if you bring in some takeaway food to eat in your room. They usually have a microwave available for heating your meal — just look at the information folder or ask at reception to find out where it is (microwaves are often located with the washing machines, dryers and vending machines — the last offering soft drinks, tea/coffee, beer and some gluten-free alcoholic options like gin and tonics and vodka or whiskey highballs).

Photo Page 25: Typical hotel buffet breakfast

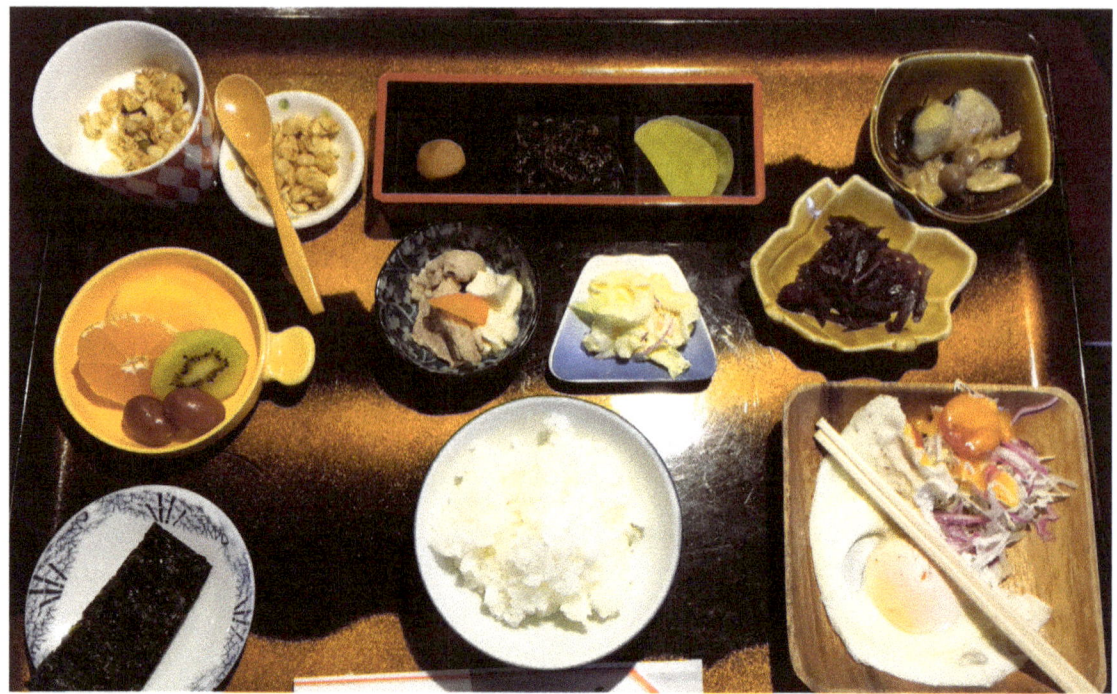

Above: Breakfast at Hotel Kinoe Sou, Kamoenai, Hokkaido

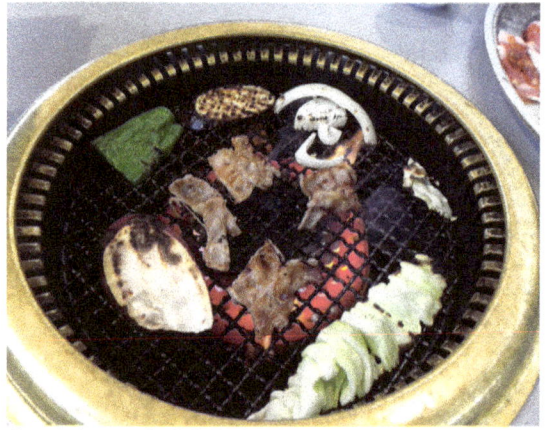

Above: Barbecue meal at Shuho Royal Hotel, Mine

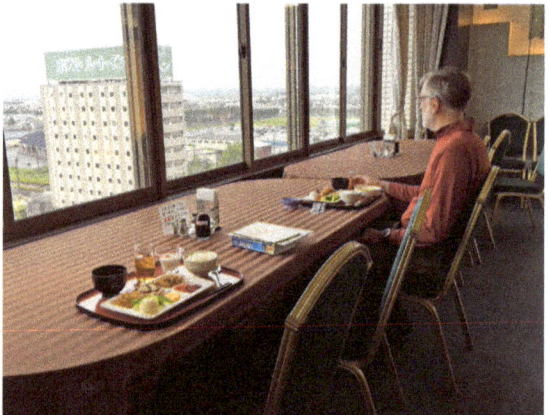

Above & Below: Typical hotel buffet breakfasts

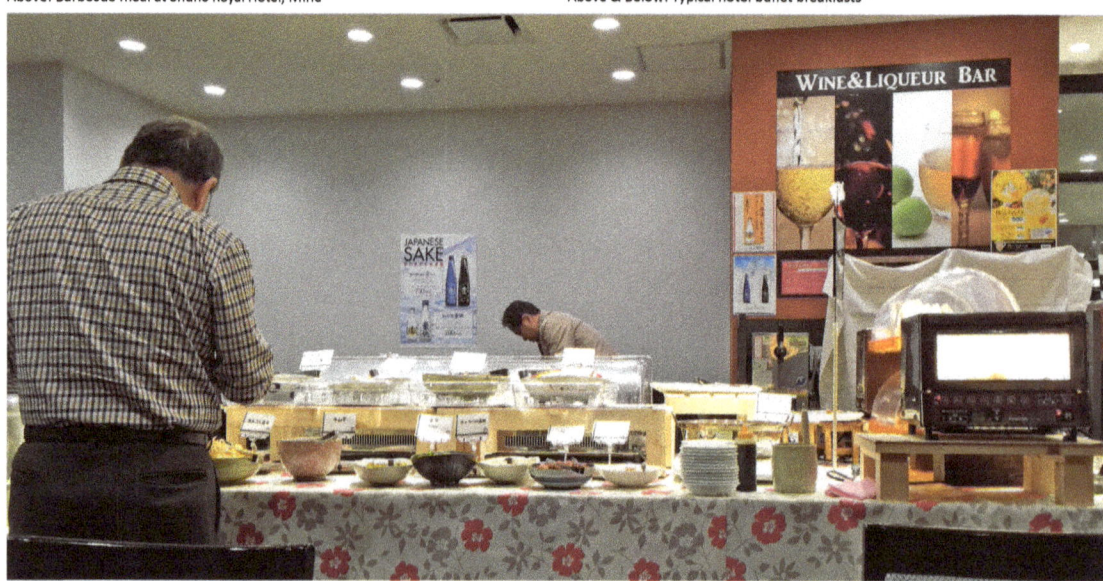

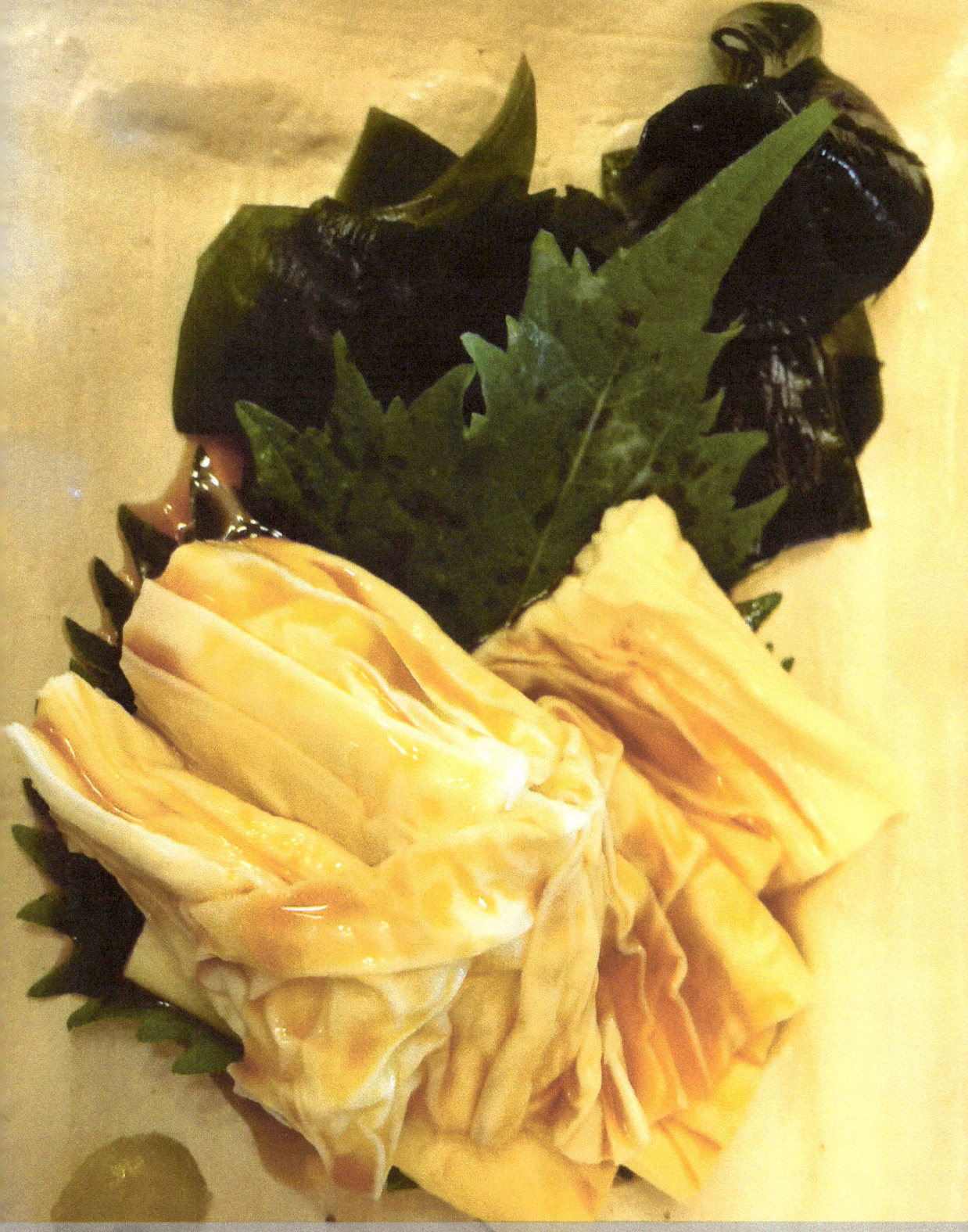

CHAPTER SIX
Other accommodation
Ryokans, Airbnbs, pensions, hostels & Youth Hostels

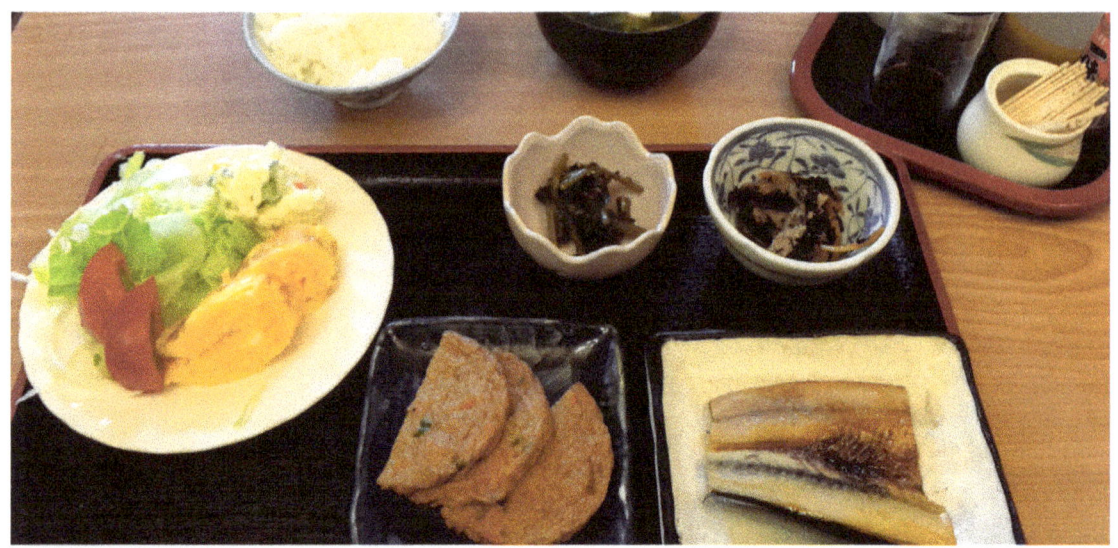

Above & Below Left: Breakfast dishes at Nikko Suginamiki Youth Hostel

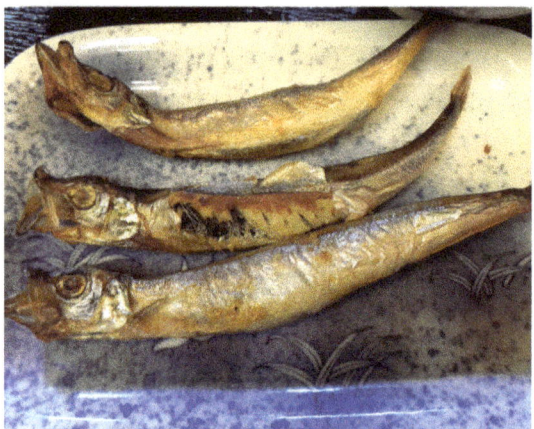

Below: Nikko Suginamiki Youth Hostel entrance

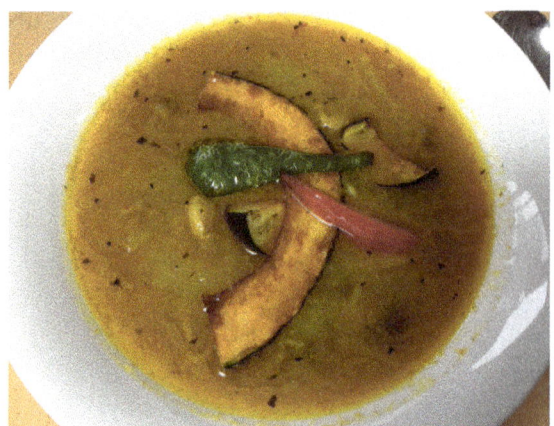

Above: Curry at Guest House Yasumizaka, Kushiro

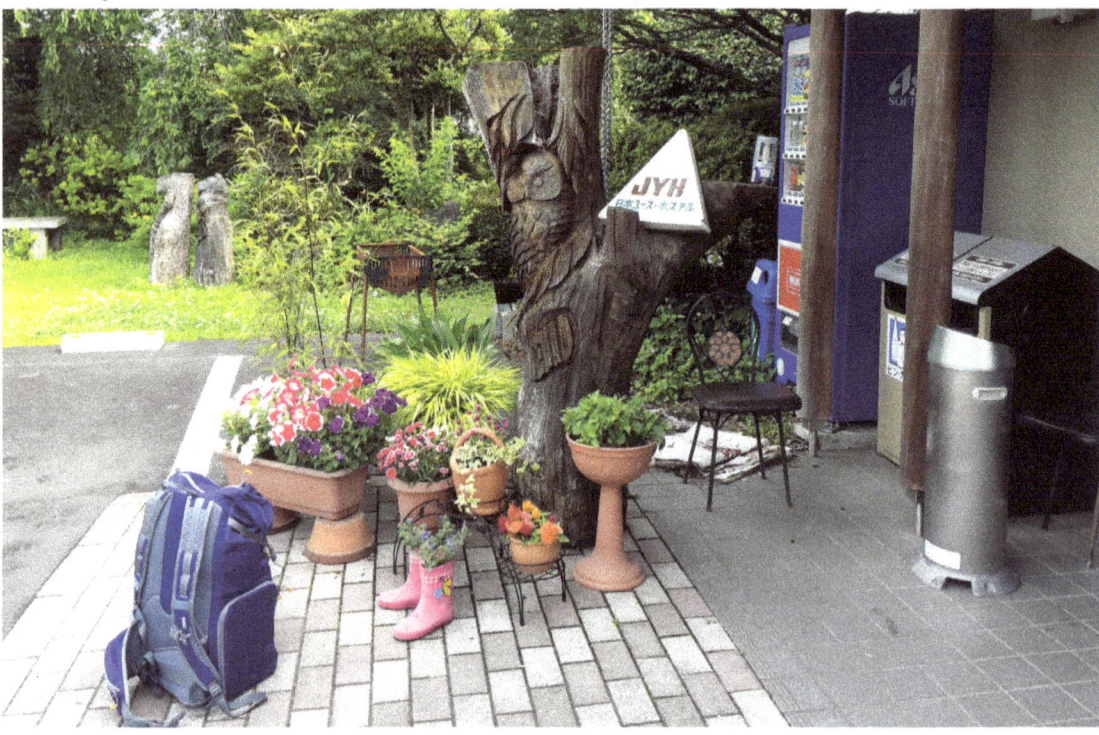

OTHER ACCOMMODATION: Ryokans, Airbnbs, pensions, hostels & Youth Hostels

Ryokans

Ryokans or Japanese inns, are traditional types of accommodation with Japanese style sleeping, on futons assembled at bedtime on a tatami (straw) floor. The room doubles as a living area during the day, with a low table and chairs or cushions that you can use for drinking tea and coffee or eating meals. Ryokans tend to be expensive but the price usually includes breakfasts and dinners, which are served either in your room or in a communal dining room. Both meals are usually quite lavish and you will need to let the host know in advance of any dietary requirements. Or, because the meals are so large, you can simply choose not to eat anything that isn't gluten-free (or swap things around with someone else). Ryokans (and hotels) usually have their own onsen or hot bath and you'll be provided with a yukata (summer dressing gown) and jacket that can be worn around the place, including the dining room. You'll also be provided with slippers to wear around after you've left your shoes at the front door. Just be very careful to change into the special slippers provided in the toilets and not to walk out of the toilets while still wearing them.

Airbnbs

Airbnbs are a great option if you want to cook your own meals. You'll find a wide variation in the type and number of cooking utensils and equipment available, from the very basic microwave, hotplate, electric jug, small fridge, crockery, cutlery, saucepan and frying pan, to very well equipped places with gorgeous crockery and all manner of appliances. Nevertheless, it's a good idea to carry your own glasses/mugs, plates, knives, forks and spoons — just in case! The nice thing about staying in Airbnbs is that they are usually located in suburbs and so give you a good idea of how Japanese people live and what's available in the local suburban shops. You'll find some ideas for cooking simple gluten-free meals in Chapter 13 (Meals at Home). And if you don't want to cook, you can simply pick up a ready-made meal from the local supermarket on your way home and eat it watching TV!

Photo Page 29: Yuba (soymilk skin) at the Nikko Suginamiki Youth Hostel

Pensions & Hostels

Pensions are usually located in out-of-the way places and have meals available. Two pensions we found had exceptional food — the That Sounds Good Jazz Pension at Tazawako, and the Pension Arumeria at Wakkanai in Hokkaido.

Hostels and guest houses are usually located smack bang in the middle of tourist destinations, and have small bedrooms but large common areas and shared cooking facilities for guests. We stayed at quite a few K's House hostels in Honshu. K's is a chain of excellent, clean hostels with friendly staff who speak a variety of languages. You can store labelled food in communal fridges and cook it yourself to eat at tables provided in the common lounge/dining room. The facilities are available day and night and the kitchens and dining areas are very well equipped. Rooms range from private singles or couples to shared dorm-style accommodation. K's staff will help you with sightseeing and transport tips and sometimes organise group outings for guests. K's House hostels are located in very convenient areas of cities such as Hiroshima, Kyoto, Tokyo (two), Takayama, Hakone, and more.

Another excellent hostel we used was Grids in Sapporo, which offers breakfasts for a reasonable price — but which aren't gluten-free. Hostels usually hold regular social functions where you can meet other travellers. While they are usually pasta or pizza type functions, you can always eat your own food.

Youth Hostels

Youth Hostels provide both private and dorm accommodation at reasonable prices. The only drawbacks are that they may be closed to guests in the middle of the day, and they are often in remote locations (which can actually make your visit more interesting!). Many hosts will, however, offer to pick you up from the nearest station. Youth hostels usually have breakfasts and dinners available if booked beforehand. The host will provide simple, wholesome meals that can be gluten-free if you explain your requirements on arrival. And you may get to try some interesting local cuisine.

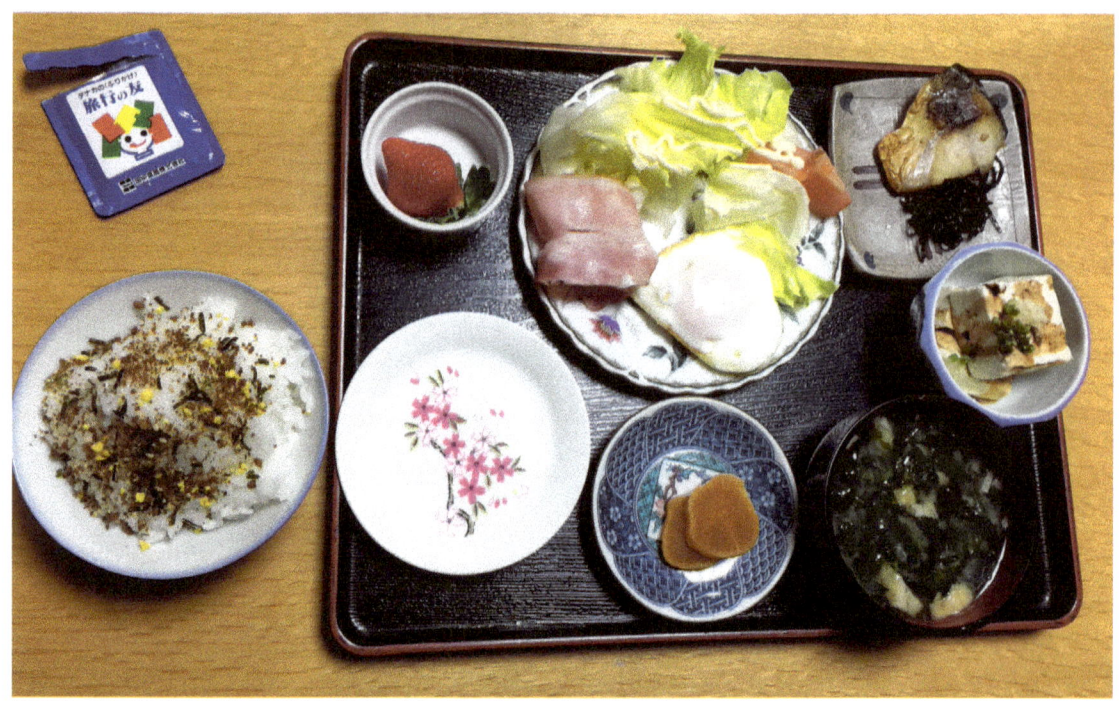

Above: Breakfast at Youth Hostel Murataya Ryokan, Takamori; Below: Dinner for two at Pension Arumeria, Wakkanai

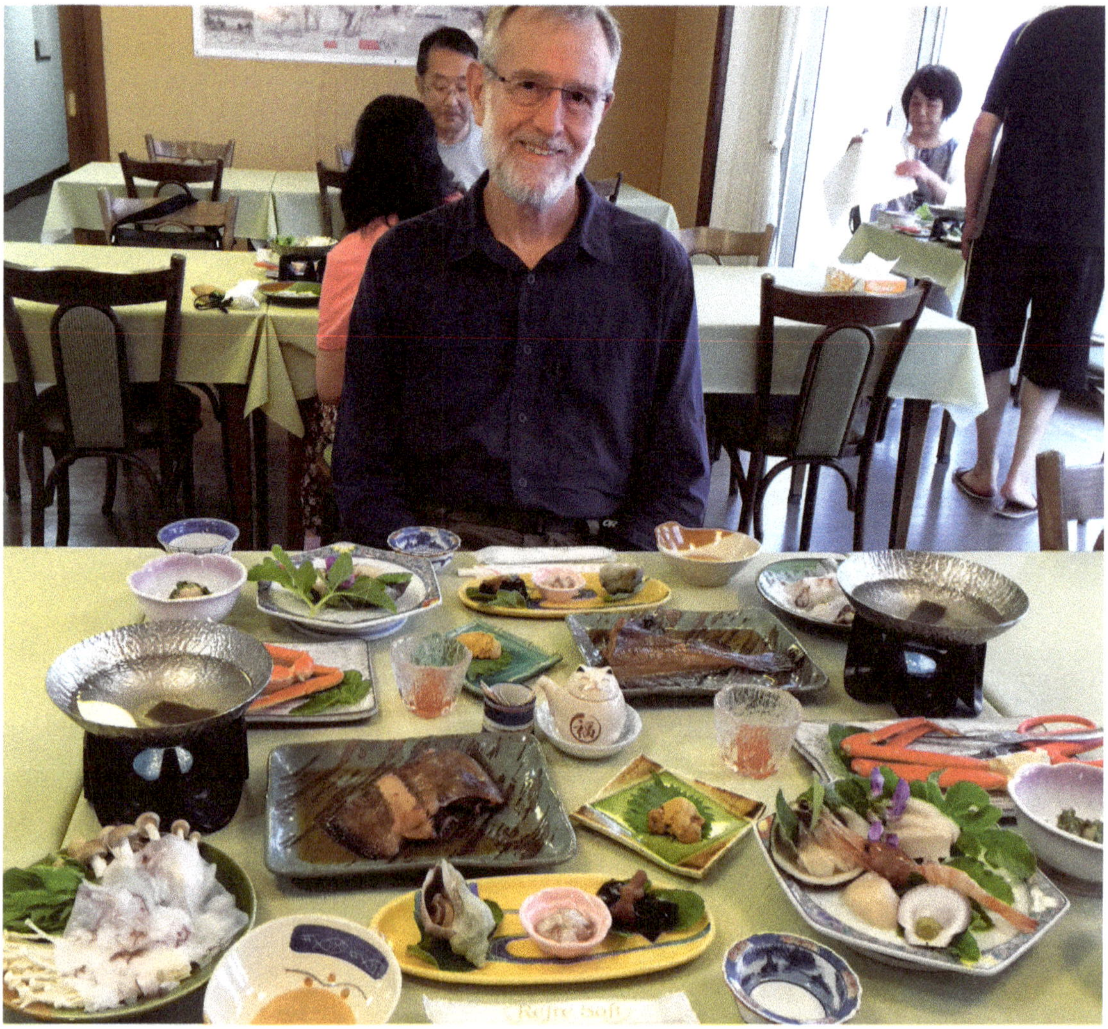

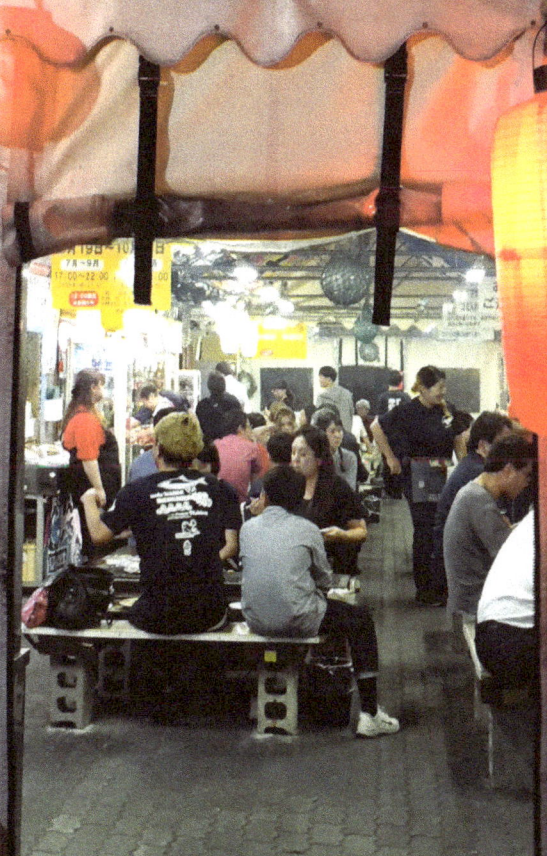

CHAPTER SEVEN

Japanese cuisine
Restaurants, teishoku, izakaya, barbecue & nabe

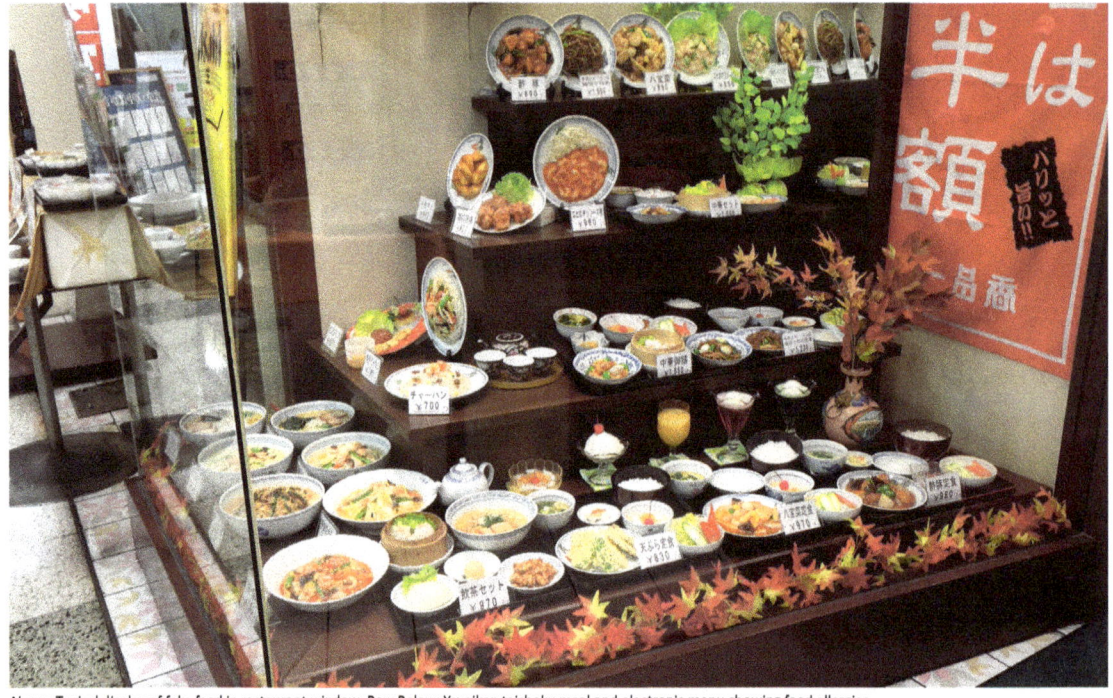

Above: Typical display of fake food in restaurant window; Row Below: Yayoiken teishoku meal and electronic menu showing food allergies

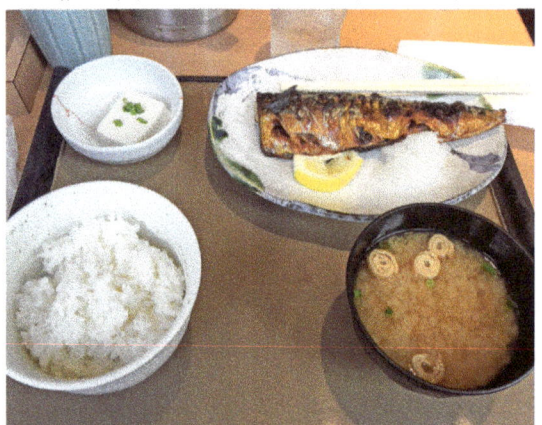
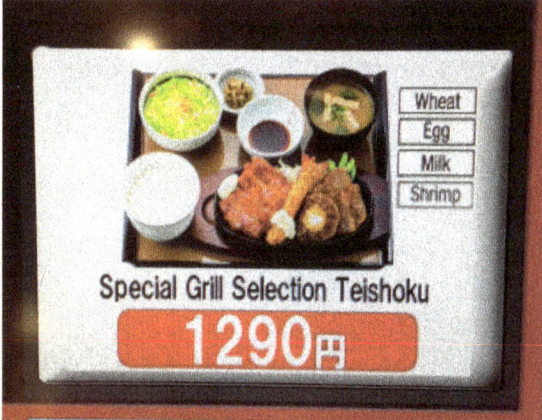

Below Left: Yakitori restaurant in Kurashiki with chicken sashimi in foreground   Below Right: Fish and rice lunch at restaurant near Ise Shrine

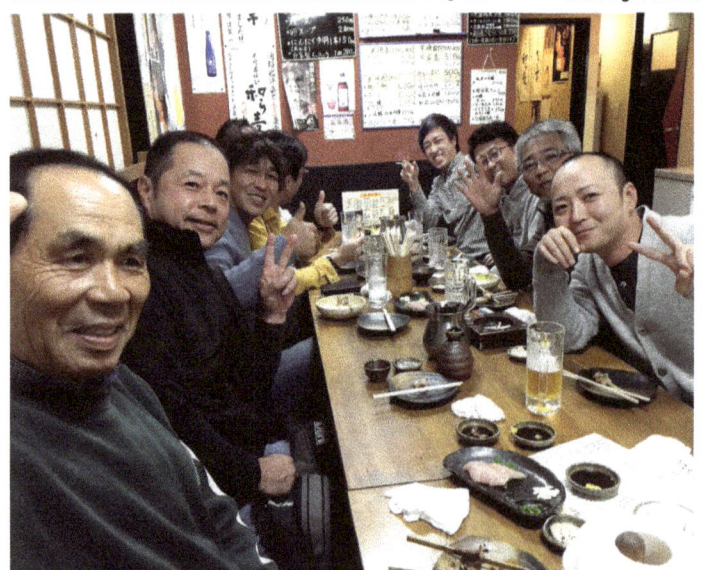
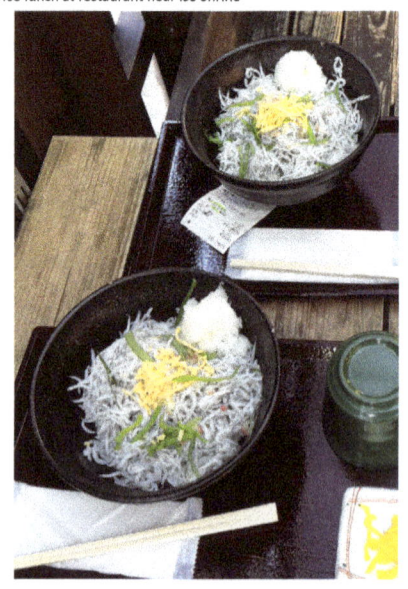

JAPANESE CUISINE: Restaurants, teishoku, izakaya, barbecue & nabe

Restaurants

Restaurants offering Japanese food come in all shapes and sizes and you'll find that in most of the touristy areas — including the areas around railway stations — most of the places have window displays of their wares. These realistic fake foods make it easy to stroll around and find the best choice of food to suit a gluten-free diet. We spent a lot of time doing this for two reasons. First, because there's often an overwhelming number of restaurants to choose from, and second, because you need to look carefully to identify what's likely to be gluten-free. The longer you spend in Japan, the more you'll hone in on what you like best out of what's available. Obviously it's wise to start with meals that are fairly plain and unlikely to have soy sauce as an ingredient — steak, chicken, sushi, sashimi, eggs, salads and rice are good to begin with. Even so, if only a tiny amount of gluten will make you ill, then you should show your restaurant card and check with the waiter or the chef.

Noodles are likely to contain wheat flour, with the exception of soba noodles that are labelled 100% buckwheat. These are rather hard to come by and will be more expensive. Rice bowls (donburi) with seafood or meat toppings can be a safe bet for coeliacs (but best to check!).

Restaurants often specialise in particular types of food. For example, we came across a small restaurant that only served steaks of different types ('yakiniku'). It only held about half a dozen people, standing, at any one time. They did manage to find some vegetables for me (a non-red-meat eater), but we had to go on to another restaurant to finish our meal. 'Yakitori' (chicken) restaurants are great for coeliacs. As long as you specify salted chicken skewers, they won't have soy sauce on them. But beware of the types of chicken on offer as you may not like the thought of chicken hearts, skin, gizzards or worse. The only meal we really didn't enjoy was called 'charcoal chicken' and it tasted just like the name. Beware too of chicken sashimi (raw) as it is served in some regions. We tried some in Kurashiki but with some trepidation. Likewise for blowfish!

You're likely to come across a range of interesting restaurants with some very unusual foods as you travel around in Japan. There are Japanese restaurants that serve whale meat. There are some with healthy/vegetarian/vegan options, and there's even the occasional gluten-free restaurant (see Chapter 20).

Teishoku

Teishoku restaurants serve meals made up of several dishes served together as a set on the same tray. Usually the set will include at least a main, rice, pickles and soup. Such meals are great value and one teishoku chain in particular (Yayoiken), with restaurants all over Japan, lists any likely allergy-causing ingredients on the electronic menu that you order from as you enter the restaurant.

Sushi train restaurants are also good value and provide a good source of gluten-free food. At Hamazushi restaurants, which are popular right around the country, you check in with a robot and order your dishes via a screen at the table. At one sushi train in Omiya near Tokyo, the dishes were delivered to each table by a model shinkansen.

Izakaya

Izakaya restaurants typically cater for groups of people wanting to party, as they provide relatively cheap dishes for sharing, along with a time-limited supply of alcohol. They are particularly popular for after-work get-togethers and tend to be a lot of fun but quite loud and sometimes smoky (yes, smoking is still allowed in restaurants in Japan).

Barbecue and nabe

Barbecue restaurants or gyu-kaku (also called robata in some areas) are a great find for gluten-free meals. The raw food of your choice — meats, vegetables, seafood — is laid out on plates so that you can cook it at your own pace on a barbecue plate or grill in the centre of your table. You can also order salads and drinks as you go. The same principle applies to nabe (hot-pot) restaurants, where there is usually a choice of 'broth' for cooking your meats and vegetables in — not all of which contain soy sauce. We particularly enjoyed soy milk nabes.

Photo Page 33: Robata (barbecue) restaurant, Kushiro

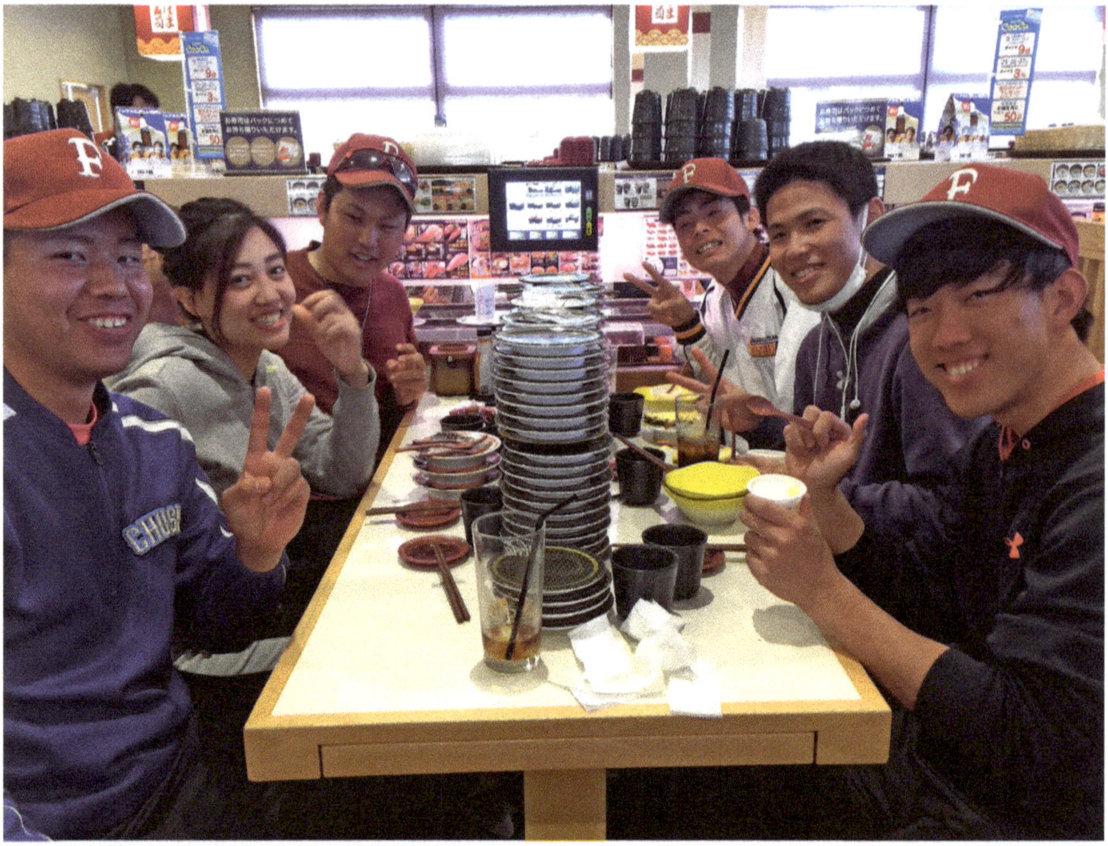

Above: Hamazushi sushi restaurant; Below: Barbecue restaurant, Tsuruoka

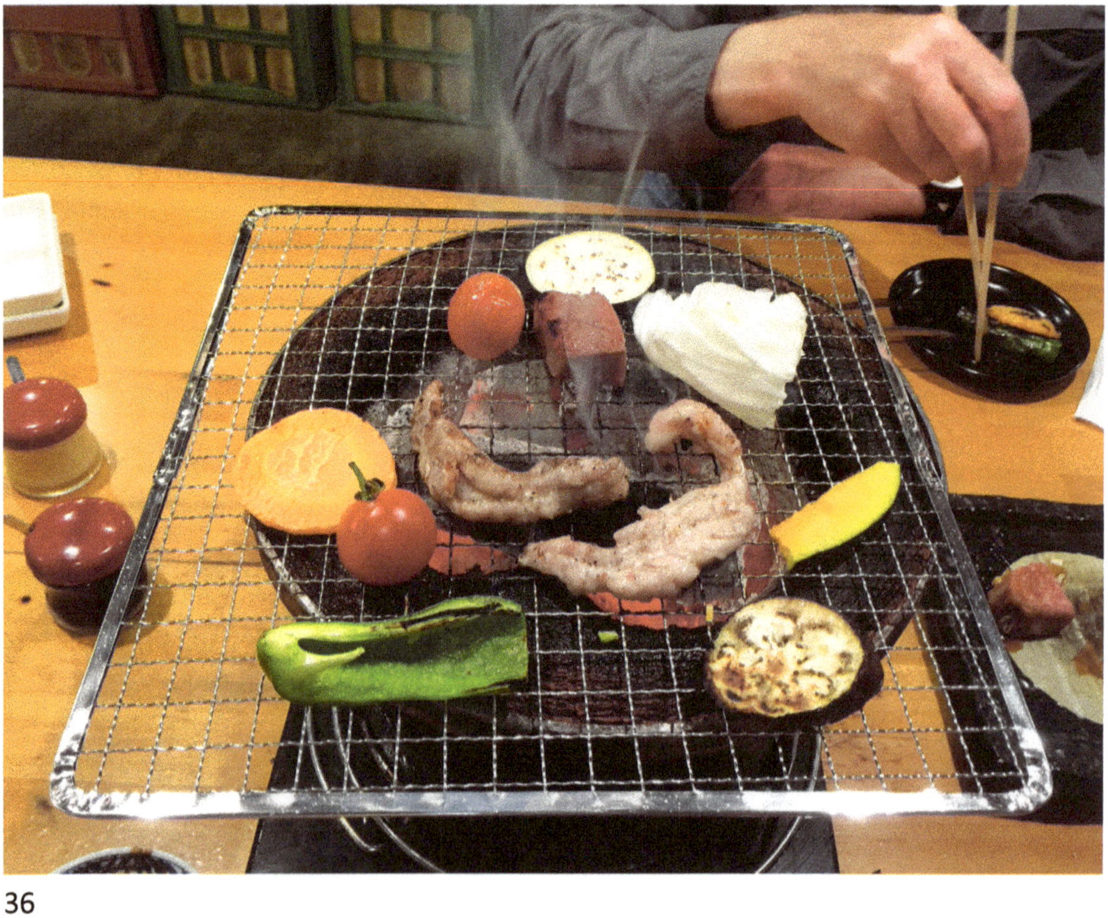

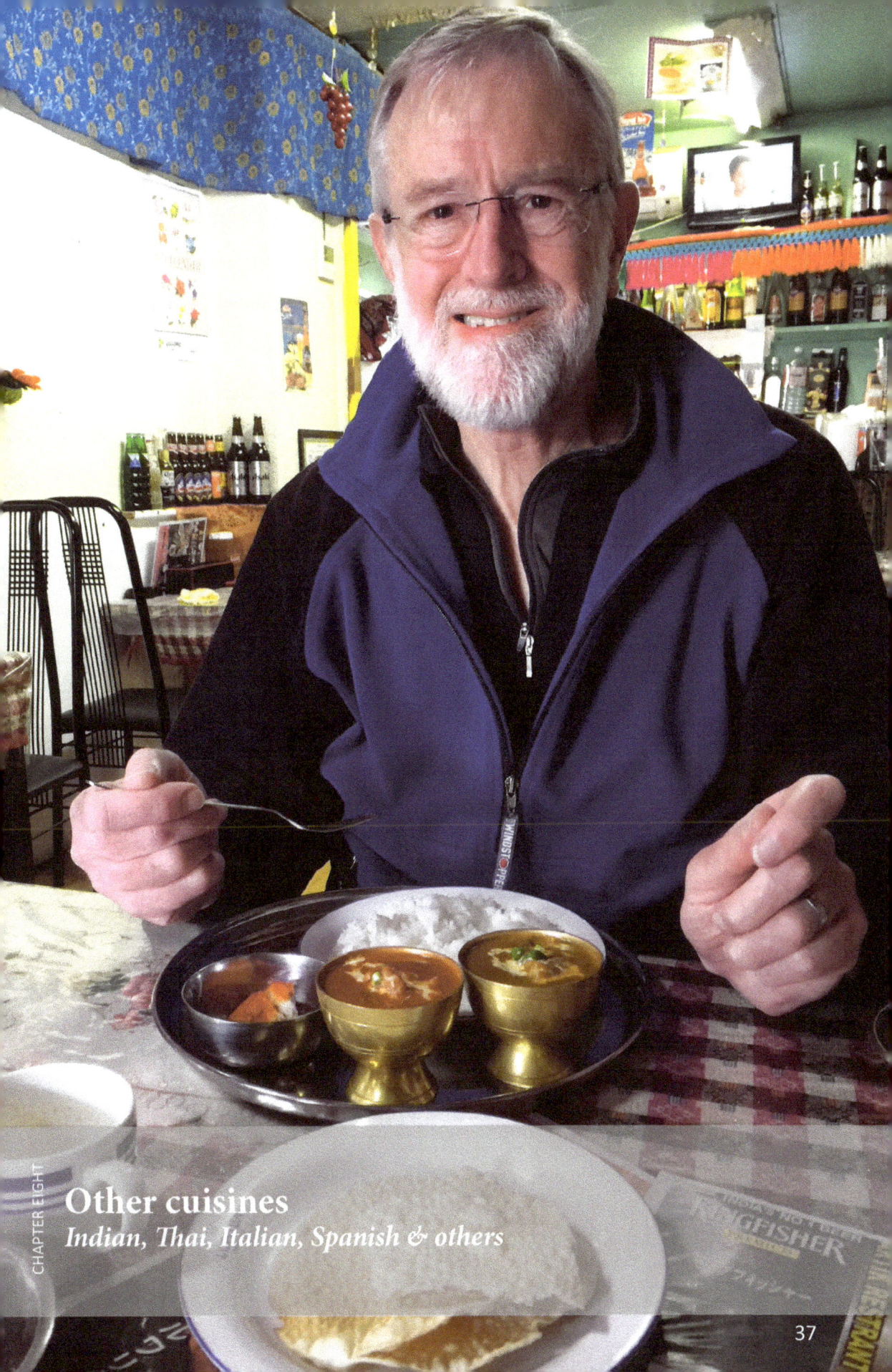

Other cuisines
Indian, Thai, Italian, Spanish & others

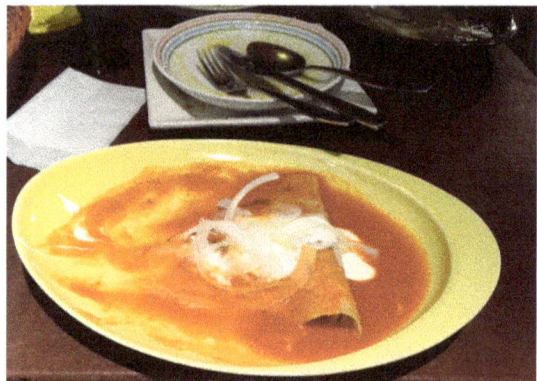

Above: Mexican restaurant in Fukuoka; Below: Pad Thai at Thai restaurant, Kyoto

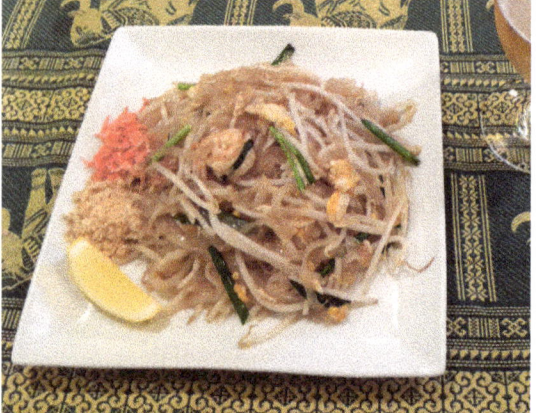

Below: Paella lunch at Spanish restaurant in Sapporo

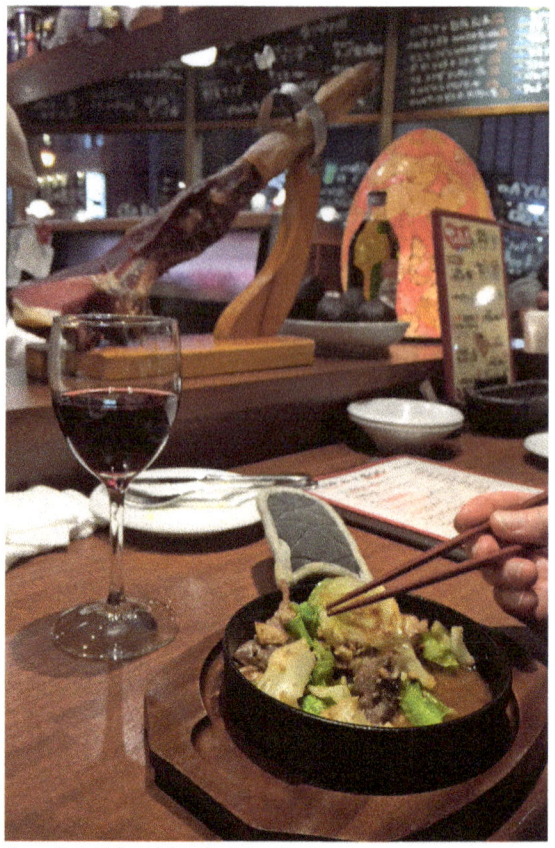

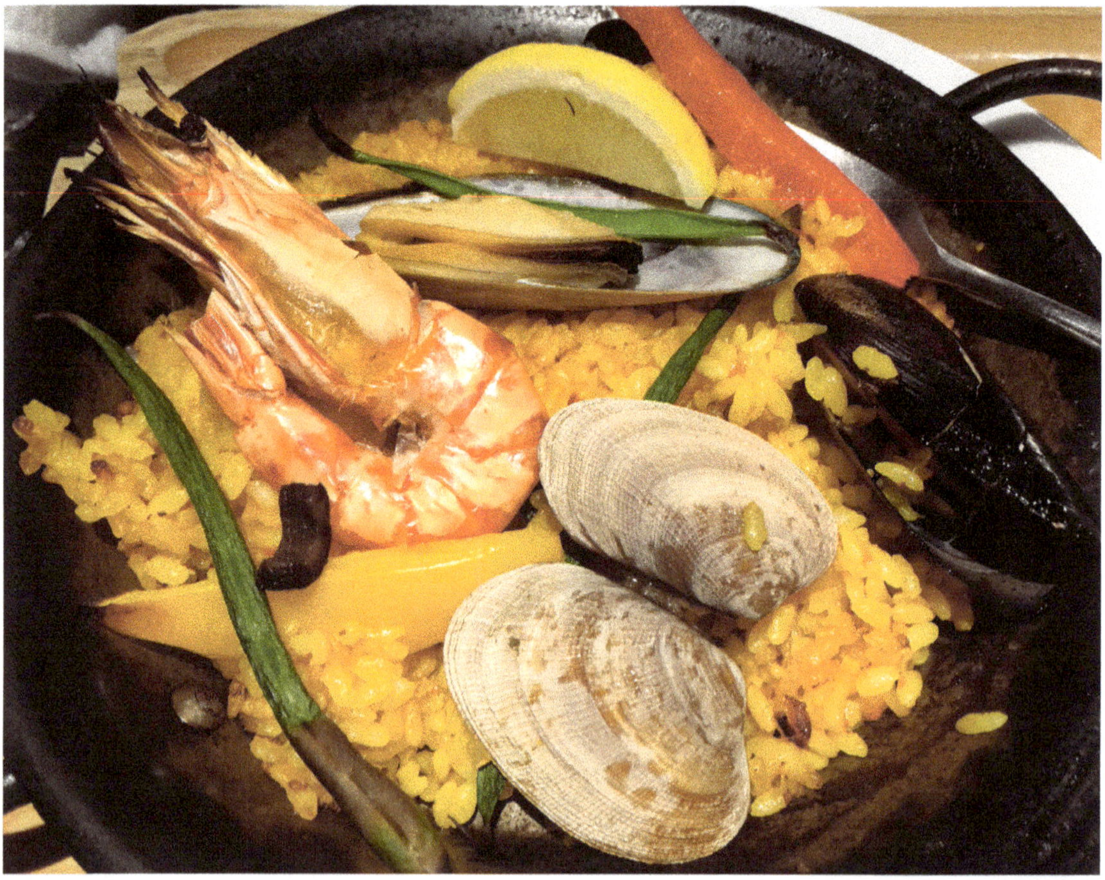

Above: Dinner at Spanish tapas bar in Susukino, Sapporo

OTHER CUISINES: Indian, Thai, Italian, Spanish & others

Indian

There are plenty of Indian and Nepalese restaurants in Japan, mostly in the major centres but also in some unexpected places. These restaurants are a particularly good choice for coeliacs because most of the dishes are made with non wheat-based flours like chick-pea or rice flour — apart from naan breads, which can always be substituted with pappadams (which are made from chick pea flour). Unlike in other parts of the world, you'll find that Japanese rice is used, rather than basmati, as it seems that foreign rice varieties aren't easy or economical to import.

Indian restaurants tend to be rather pricey for dinner. However, they usually have lunch specials in the middle of the day and these are really great value — one or two curries, with salad and a choice of rice or naan bread, as well as a drink (e.g. lassi or even beer). We found that many Indian restaurants offered a very economical 'ladies' lunch special' that men were not entitled to order. The curries in Indian restaurants are much the same as you'd find in other parts of the world — butter chicken, lamb korma, and so on, with the usual accompaniments. For companions of coeliacs, the huge naan breads are exceptionally good.

Thai

Thai restaurants tend to proliferate in the larger touristy cities only, such as Kyoto and Tokyo. Though not as cheap as Japanese restaurants at dinner time, the food is good and seems authentic. As with Indian restaurants, you'll be served Japanese medium grain rice rather than jasmine rice. However, Thai food features rice noodles which are gluten-free and thus suitable for coeliacs. We found our usual favourites, spicy baked whole fish and pad thai, which were always good.

Italian

Italian restaurants are everywhere in Japan, and seem to be very popular with Japanese people, especially pizza and pasta places. These are, of course, rarely suitable for coeliacs and therefore these restaurants are best avoided. If you do happen to be in an Italian restaurant the best bet is to look for a risotto as these are generally gluten-free.

Spanish

Spanish restaurants can be found in the major Japanese cities or tourist areas. They generally offer cheap paellas at lunchtime. These are individual hot plates of spicy rice with seafood, chicken and some vegetables. They are good winter warmers when you can't eat the ubiquitous noodle dishes (ramen and udon), but are also good at any time. Like Indian, Thai and Italian restaurants, Spanish places are far more expensive at night for dinner, although there seems to be a trend towards Spanish tapas bars, which offer small share plates to have with drinks. You're sure to find some dishes that are gluten-free — at a price!

Others

The few Mexican restaurants we came across had some good choices that were gluten-free — such as corn chips, guacamole, corn tacos, etc. However, they were quite expensive for small amounts. There seem to be quite a number of French restaurants in the major cities, however we only tried one — because it was the venue chosen to farewell one of our classmates. There were some meat cold cuts and vegetable dishes that were gluten-free, as well as some particularly delicious gelatos for dessert, but predictably most dishes were unsuitable for coeliacs. The most noticeable French influence is the sheer number of French style bakeries throughout Japan, including in supermarkets — not really suitable sources of food for coeliacs!

There's an increasing American influence on the fast food cuisine in Japan. However, if you travel to Okinawa in the south, where the American military bases are located, you'll find a strange well-established fusion of American and Japanese cuisines. Dishes such as taco rice and stir fry with spam (precooked pork in half a dozen or more different flavours) are gluten-free and very popular. The Okinawan cuisine is particularly healthy because of its staple purple vegetables — such as 'beni-imo' (purple sweet potato).

Photo Page 37: Lunch at Indian restaurant in Kyoto

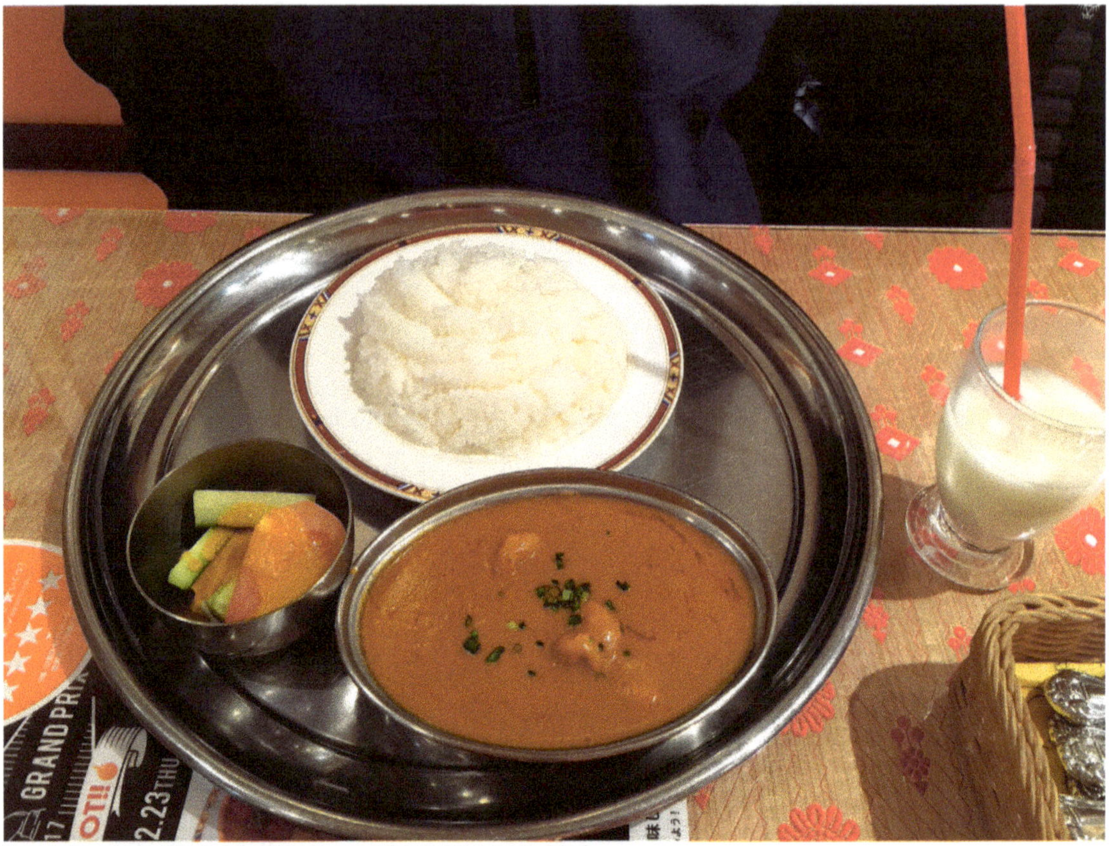

Above: Indian restaurant Fukuoka; Below: Vegetable curry at Camp Hakata restaurant, Fukuoka

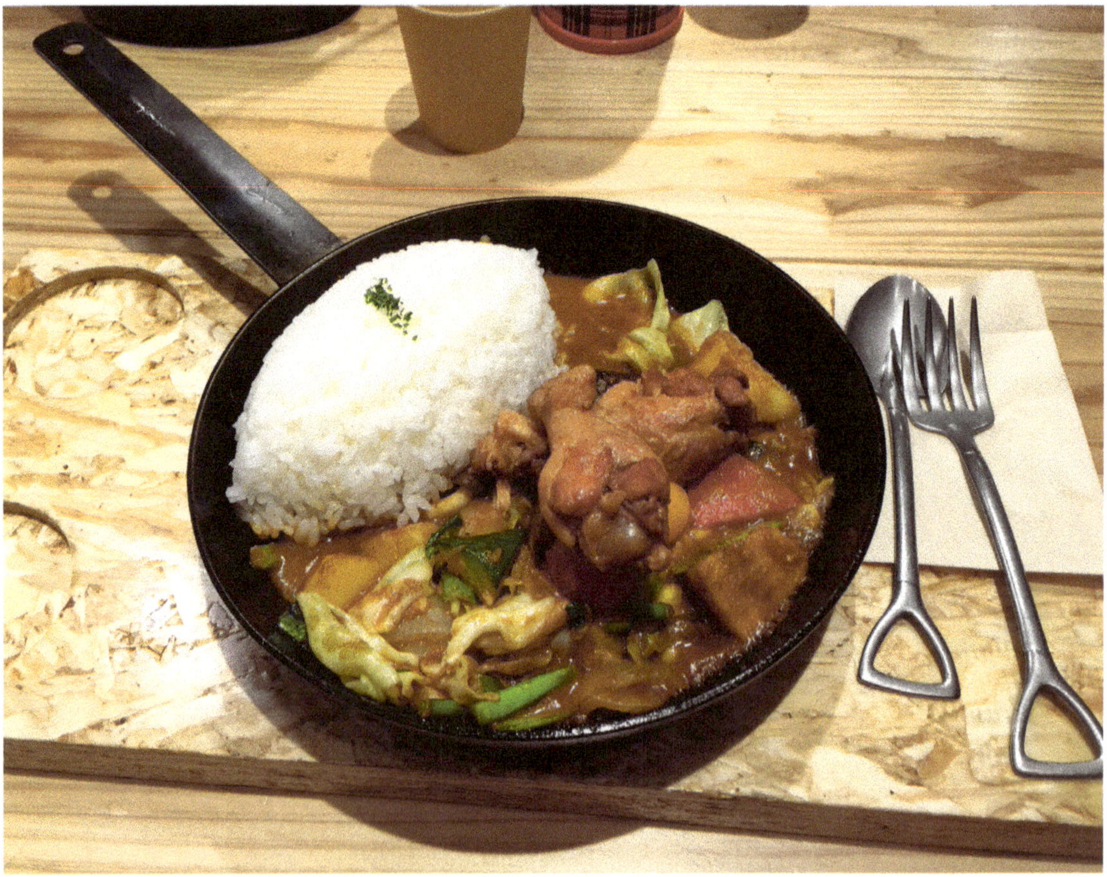

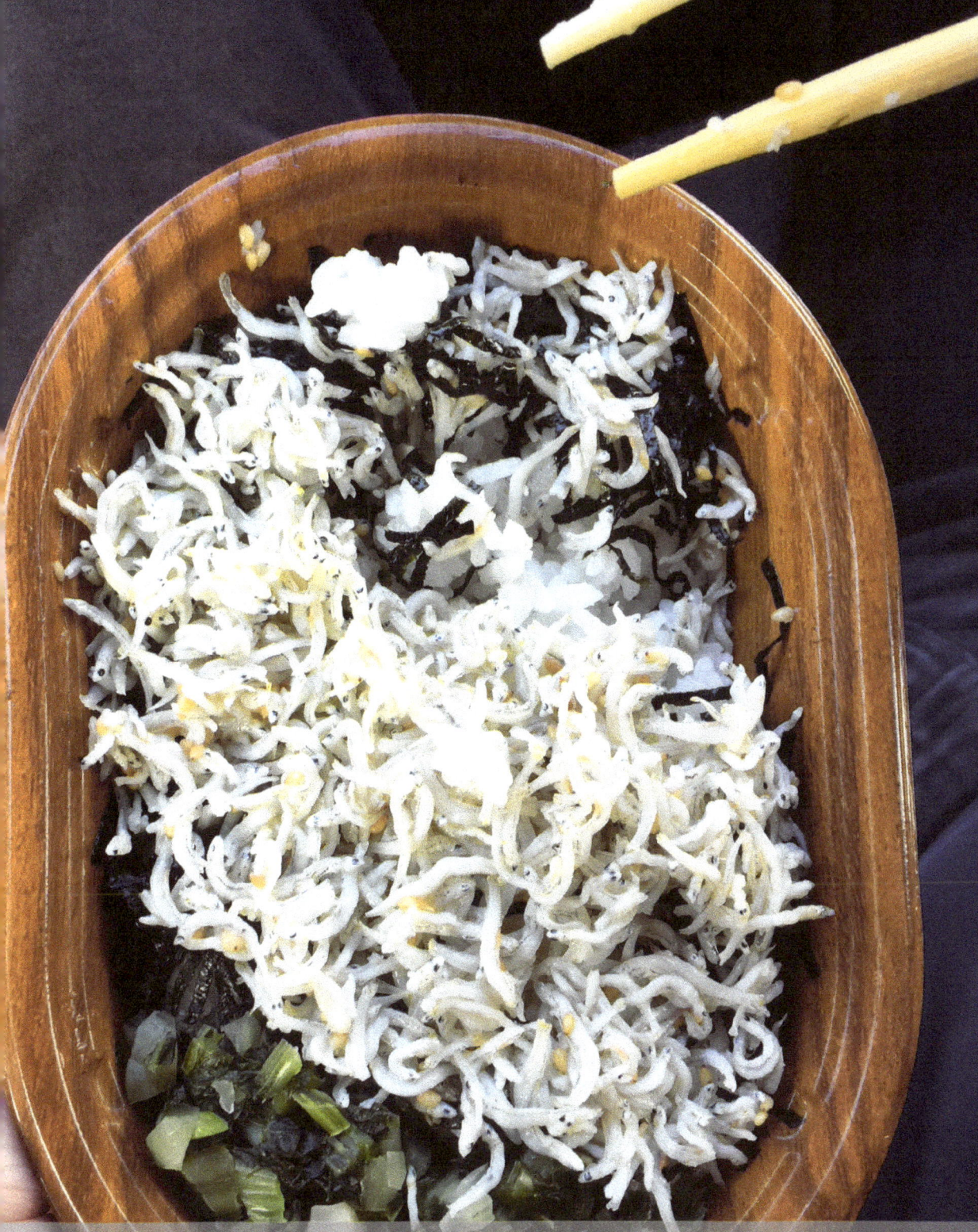

CHAPTER NINE

Takeaways
Convenience stores, supermarkets & railway stations

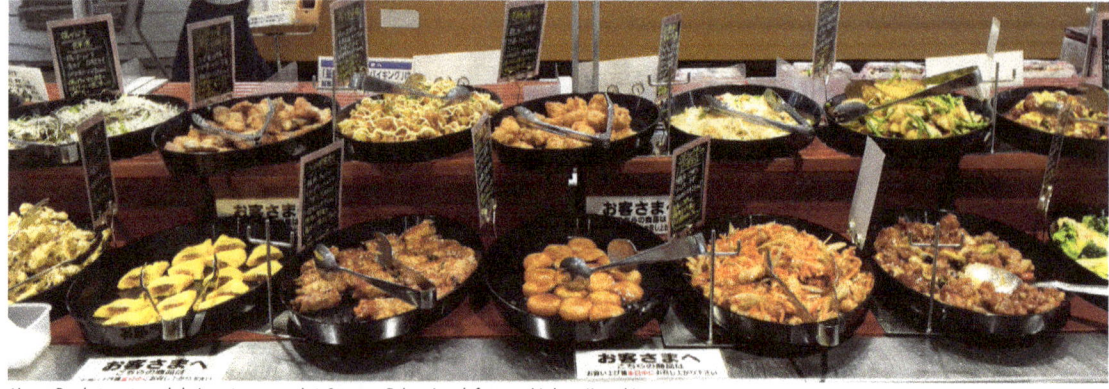
Above: Ready-to-eat meal choices at supermarket, Sapporo; Below: Lunch from sushi shop, Kagoshima

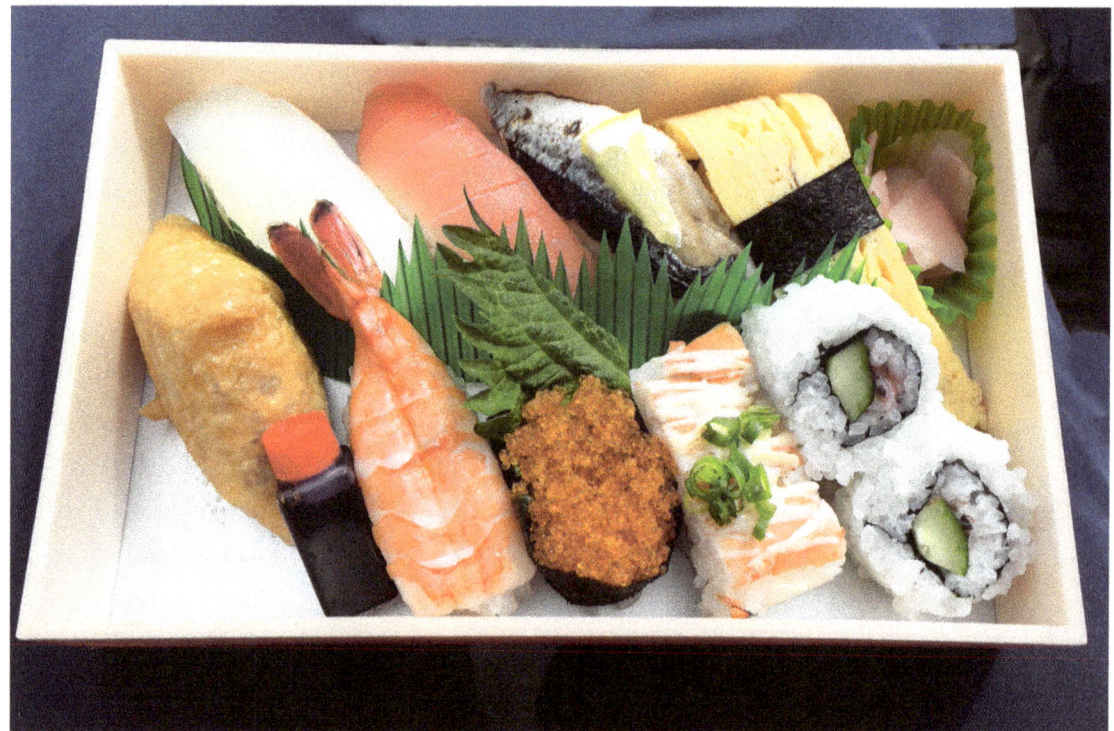

Below Left: Sashimi and salads from local supermarket, Hakodate; Below Right: Hot vegetable rice takeaway bentos, Kumamoto Station

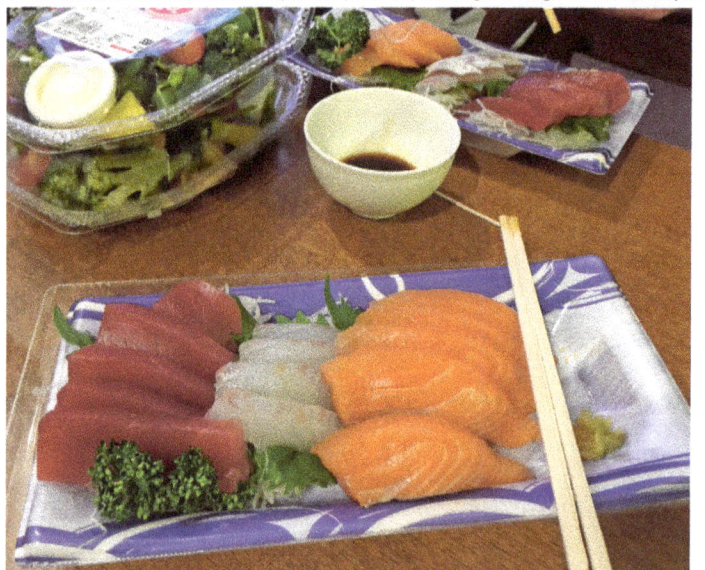
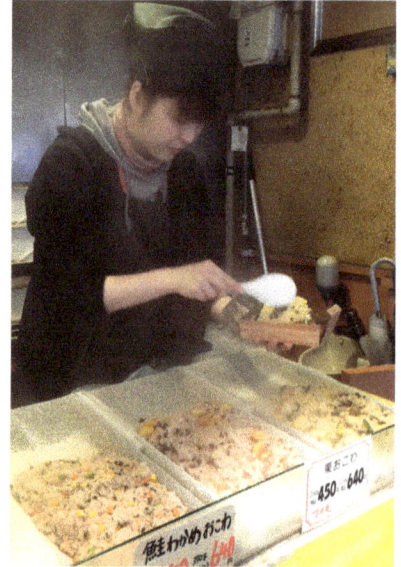

TAKEAWAYS: Convenience stores, supermarkets & railway stations

Convenience stores

Convenience stores — Seven Eleven, Lawson Station, Family Mart, Aeon Mini and others — are an absolute godsend for coeliacs. If there are no restaurants nearby or nothing gluten-free in the only small supermarket in town, then head to a convenience store, or 'konbini'. They are everywhere, even in the countryside, and you're sure to find something nice to eat. Not only that, you'll be able to pick up all sorts of other items, such as towels, alcohol, batteries, etc. Particular regions might have mostly one chain of konbini, but they all stock a similar range of foods and goods. Nevertheless, you'll soon come to prefer certain items at one particular brand of store.

The best thing about konbinis is that they sell whole meals. These are especially good for fresh, filling and nutritious lunches on the go, and dinners when you don't want to cook. While you'll find a lot of the usual suspects in convenience stores — sandwiches, noodles, pasta, breads and cakes — there are usually at least some gluten-free options, such as donburi (rice bowls), sashimi, sushi and salads, as well as bento boxes (meat/fish plus pickles, rice and other things — see below) and onigiri (savoury rice balls with a range of fillings).

Because Japan has such a large population, the turnover of these popular meals is very rapid, so the only catch for finding your favourite gluten-free meal is that the convenience store may have sold out of them. Disappointingly, this was the case sometimes with the Lawson Station grilled salmon onigiri, which became our favourites. If suitable whole meals aren't available, then don't despair, you'll probably be able to find a bunch of ingredients that you can use to assemble a meal — such as individually packaged pieces of chicken and other meats, hard boiled eggs, salted yakitori (chicken skewers), sealed bags of potato salad, pumpkin salad, 'edamame' (soy beans cooked in the pod), and so on.

Meals can be picked up at convenience stores 24/7 and taken home, or many stores have tables and chairs so that you can eat in. The staff will microwave the meals for you and cutlery and serviettes are provided, along with hot water (intended for hydrating cup noodles, but can also be used for drinks). Sometimes, when you're out and about, it's handy to have somewhere comfortable and sheltered to eat lunch, at a place where there are toilets available.

Supermarkets

Takeaway meals are also available in most supermarkets but be careful to look along both left and right sides, as well as along the back wall, because the sushi and sashimi are often in a separate area from the salads and fried foods. Besides sushi and sashimi, large supermarkets (and department stores) also usually stock a wide range of prepared meals, including bento boxes (see below), yakitori (chicken skewers), and many fried and deep fried, breadcrumbed or battered (tempura) fish, meat and vegetables. Note that only the salted yakitori will be gluten-free, and you'll need to avoid most of the other grilled or fried food. Have a good look though, as you may find some dishes that are gluten-free, such as omelettes or fish and vegetable patties. You'll also find a myriad of nibbles and snacks, drinks and sweets in supermarkets and convenience stores.

Railway stations

If you're wanting something substantial to eat for breakfast, lunch or dinner on a long distance train trip, you'll find a range of eki bento (station bento boxes) at the major train stations and on board some of the shinkansens. Some stations and shopping areas also have stalls selling various hot rice mixtures, which are great winter warmers for breakfasts while waiting for a train. There should be pictures or models displayed at the bento stall showing what's inside the brightly packaged bentos. If a bento has one or two small items that you suspect aren't gluten-free then you simply have to discard those or give them to a friend, and eat the rest. In regional areas, you might even be lucky enough to pick up a bento box featuring local specialties — such as the vegetarian sushi and the seared bonito sashimi in Shikoku.

Photo Page 41: Takeaway fish and rice meal from convenience store

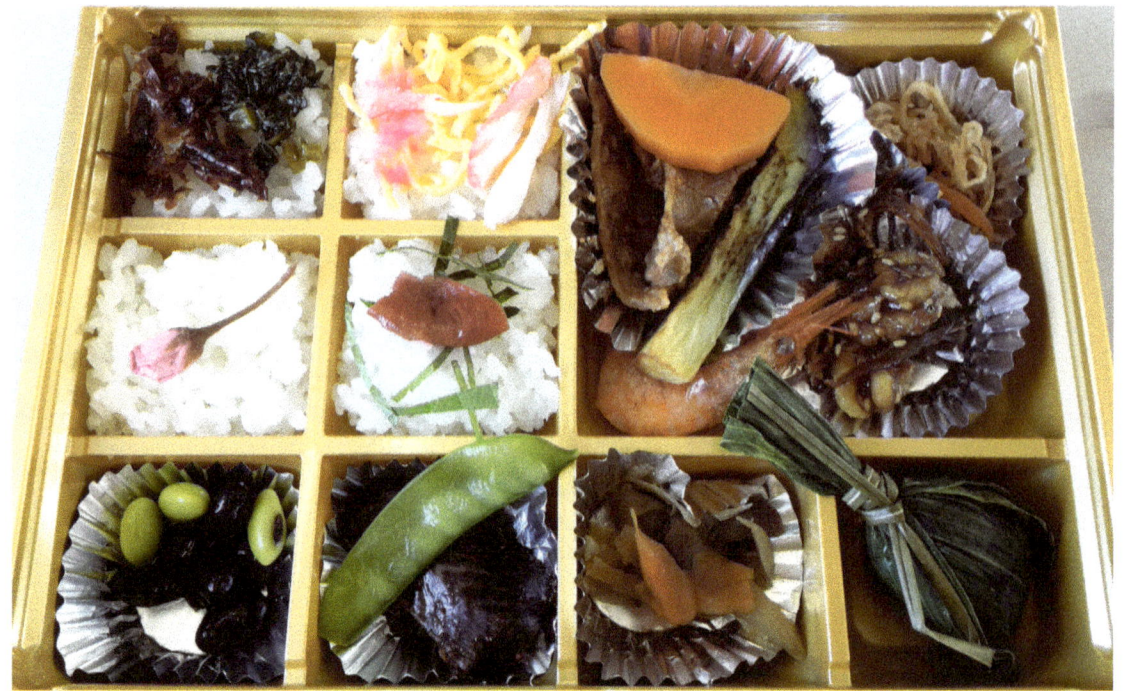
Above: Eki bento box on Shinkansen

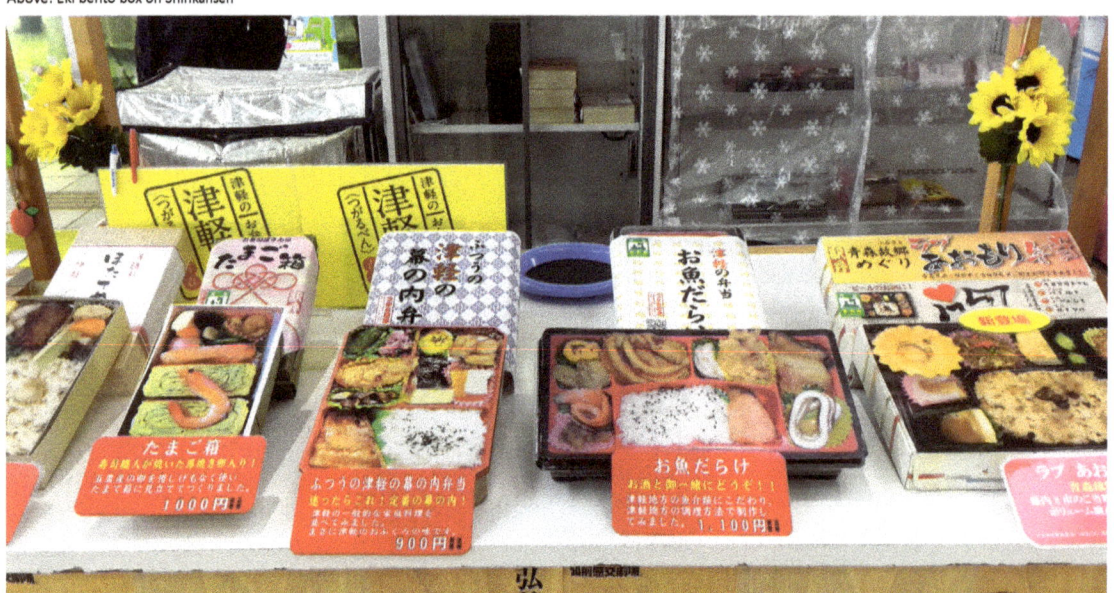
Above: Eki bentos at Shinkansen station; Below: Eki bento box on Shinkansen

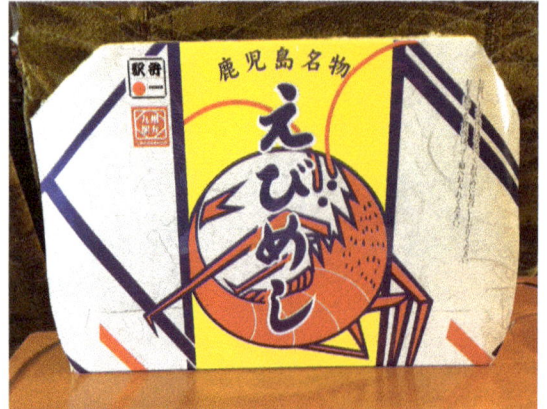
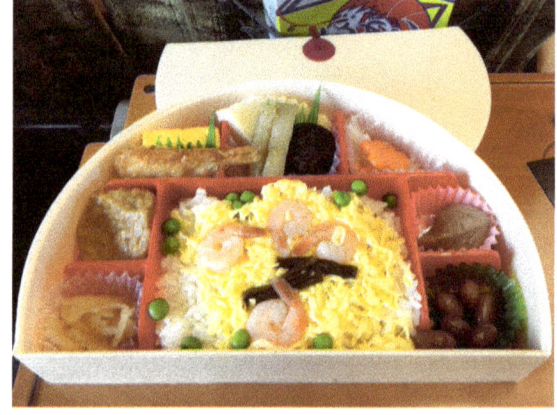

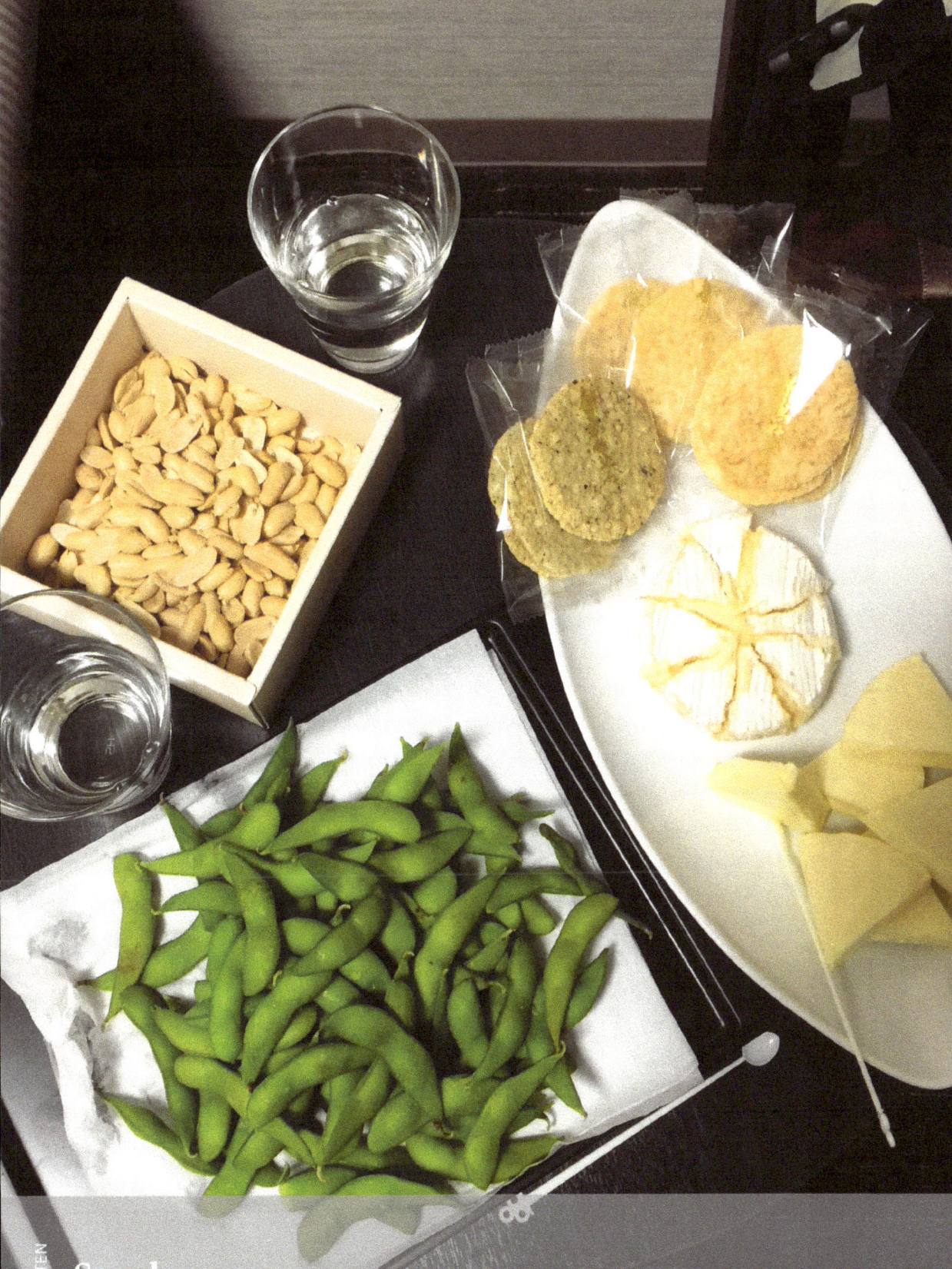

Snacks
Nibbles & snack foods

CHAPTER TEN

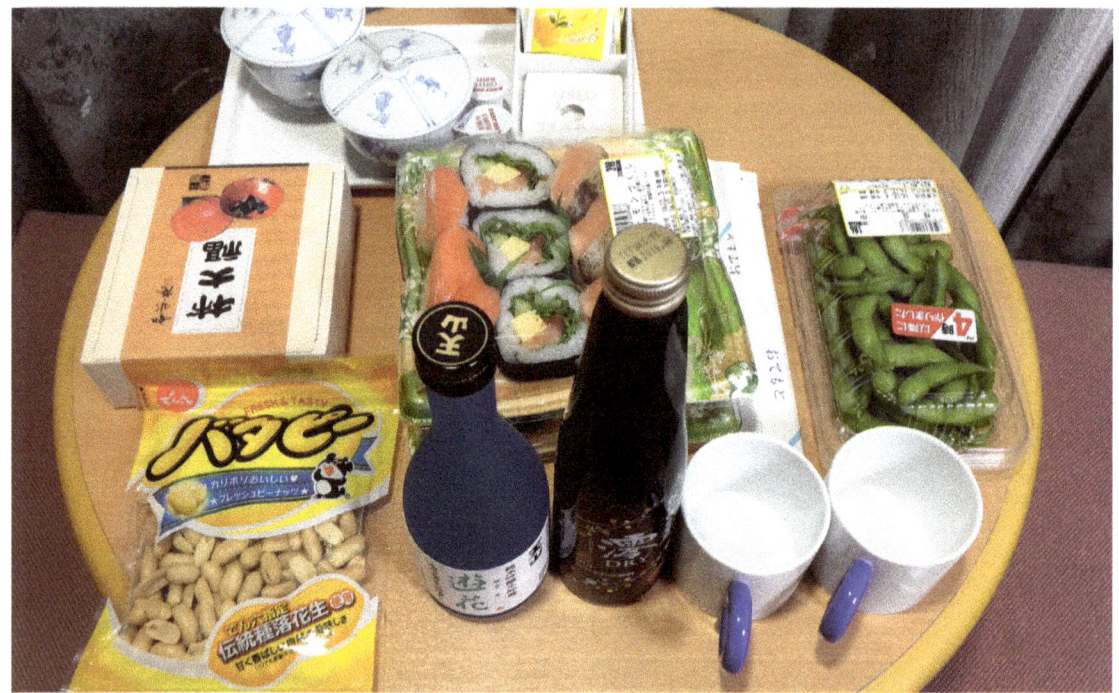

Above: Snacks, dinner, sake and sparkling sake in hotel room; Below: Salmon onigiri from convenience store

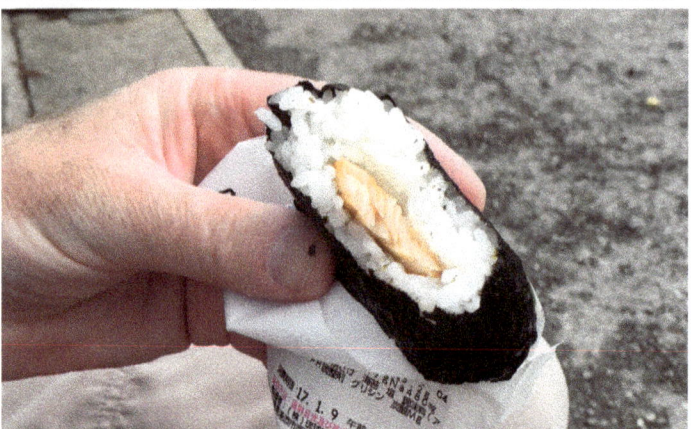

Below: Hot sweet potatoes at supermarket, Takamatsu; Right: Rice crackers from supermarket

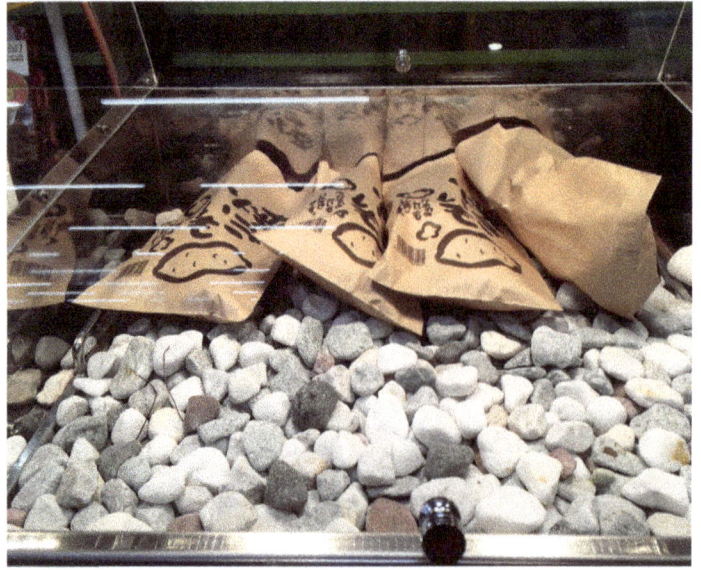

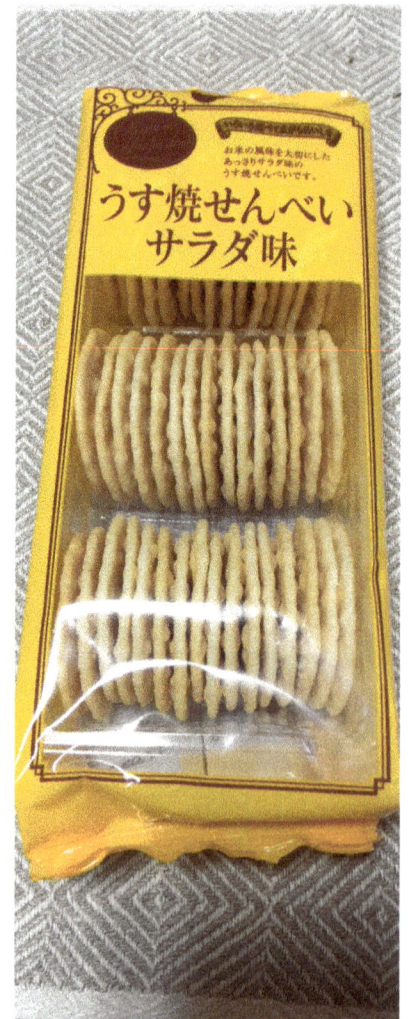

SNACKS — Nibbles & snack foods

Nibbles

If you're fond of a pre-dinner drink, then there are plenty of options for both gluten-free drinks and gluten-free nibbles. Forget about beer — gluten-free beer either doesn't exist in Japan or is very rare.

While your friends down a glass or two of great Japanese beer, you don't have to miss out. 'Sake' (rice wine) — cold varieties and warm ones — is excellent and reasonably priced and there is also a huge range of 'shochu' (distilled sake made from rice, barley or sweet potato) which is safe for coeliacs because it is distilled. Higher quality sake and sochu are, of course, more expensive. You'll also find plenty of wine and spirits are available and these are cheaper than they are in Australia.

Gluten-free nibbles to have with your drinks include nuts (peanuts are the most economical, but others such as cashews and macadamias are also common); edamame beans (bought ready-cooked at supermarkets or convenience stores or bought frozen and thawed in boiling water, just add salt; rice crackers (about 20% are wheat-free, you need to check on the packet); potato chips (not all are gluten-free, you have to read the labels); sweet potato chips; mixed vegetable chips; cherry tomatoes, sliced carrots, avocados (made into guacomole), sushi and sashimi. The purple sweet potato chips and other purple nibbles in Okinawa are particularly nice, as well as being full of healthy anti-oxidants.

Cheeses, which are gluten-free, are available in a limited range in Japan. Plain or 'camembert' (not the real thing!) are usually available in convenience stores, while more fancy types can be found in supermarkets and department stores. However, even the cheeses from Hokkaido are expensive, as are the imported (mostly French) varieties.

Snack foods

Convenience stores and larger supermarkets are particularly good sources of snack foods. Along with rice crackers, nuts, sultanas, and chips, there are plenty of sweet snacks like chocolates, lollies, ice creams and mochi available. However, the single most useful items are the Soyjoy bars.

Soyjoy bars are health bars that come in a variety of yummy flavours — such as strawberry, apple, blueberry, raisin, peanut, almond, chocolate and banana — and all are gluten-free, made from real fruit and ground whole soy. They are sold in convenience stores and supermarkets, though any one store will usually only stock two or three flavours. Soyjoys are often hard to find as they have their own special display boxes and aren't usually placed amongst similar products. Look at the ends of aisles or in other odd places, and if you can't find them, ask! Only once did we come across a packet of (six) Soyjoys in a supermarket, and a couple of times we found small versions in vending machines. Soyjoy bars have a long shelf life and are great standby foods for boosting your energy levels during days of sightseeing or on long walks, so it's a good idea to stock up with these gluten-free goodies when you can find them.

Onigiri — rice balls — are a delicious takeaway that are good for lunches on the go or as snacks. They come in many varieties — including grilled salmon, tuna, salmon roe, chicken, picked plum, shrimp. However, it's best to check the label to ensure the one you want contains no wheat. While onigiri are usually made from short grain white rice around a filling, and are wrapped in 'nori' seaweed, there are also onigiri with vegetables and egg scattered throughout, brown rice onigiri and unwrapped onigiri. Wrapped onigiri usually have very clever packaging that keeps the seaweed separate and thus crisp until the packet is opened. Nevertheless, they should be eaten the day they are bought. In winter, look for a stand of hot sweet potatoes in supermarkets.

Excellent stores to buy imported foods in general are Kaldi Coffee Farms. These stores can be found in the shopping malls around the railway stations of large Japanese cities. They sell cheeses, nuts and some other gluten-free snacks (and groceries in general) from outside Japan, as well as a range of coffees. They stock many of the things you may be homesick for — but at a price!

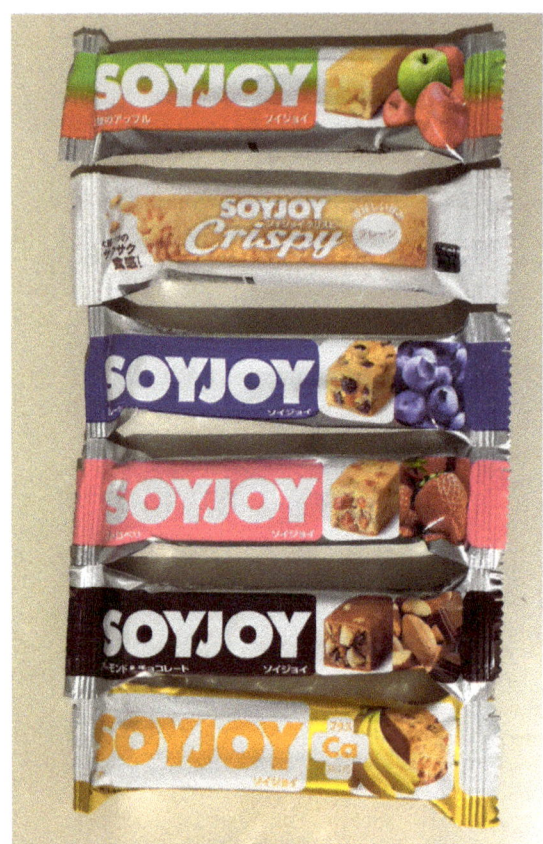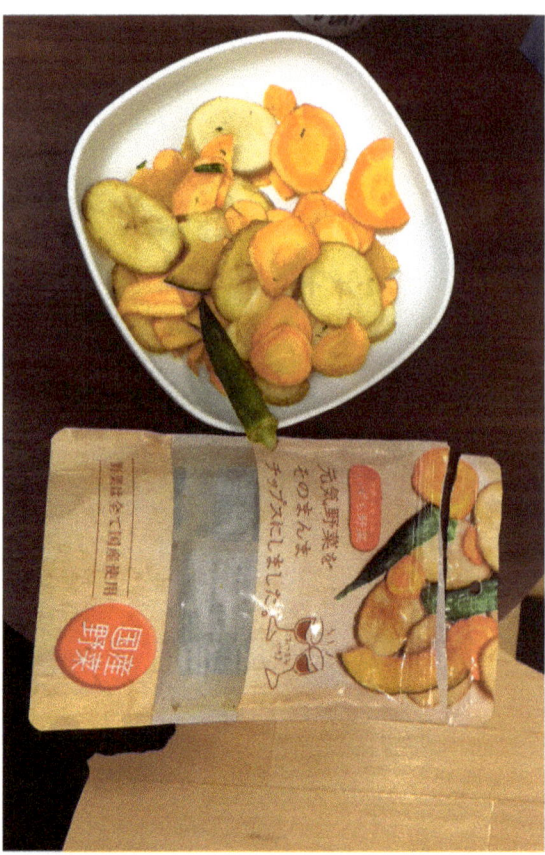

Above Left: Soyjoys from supermarket; Above Right: Freeze-dried vegetable snacks from supermarket; Below: Purple sweet potato snacks from growers' market in Okinawa

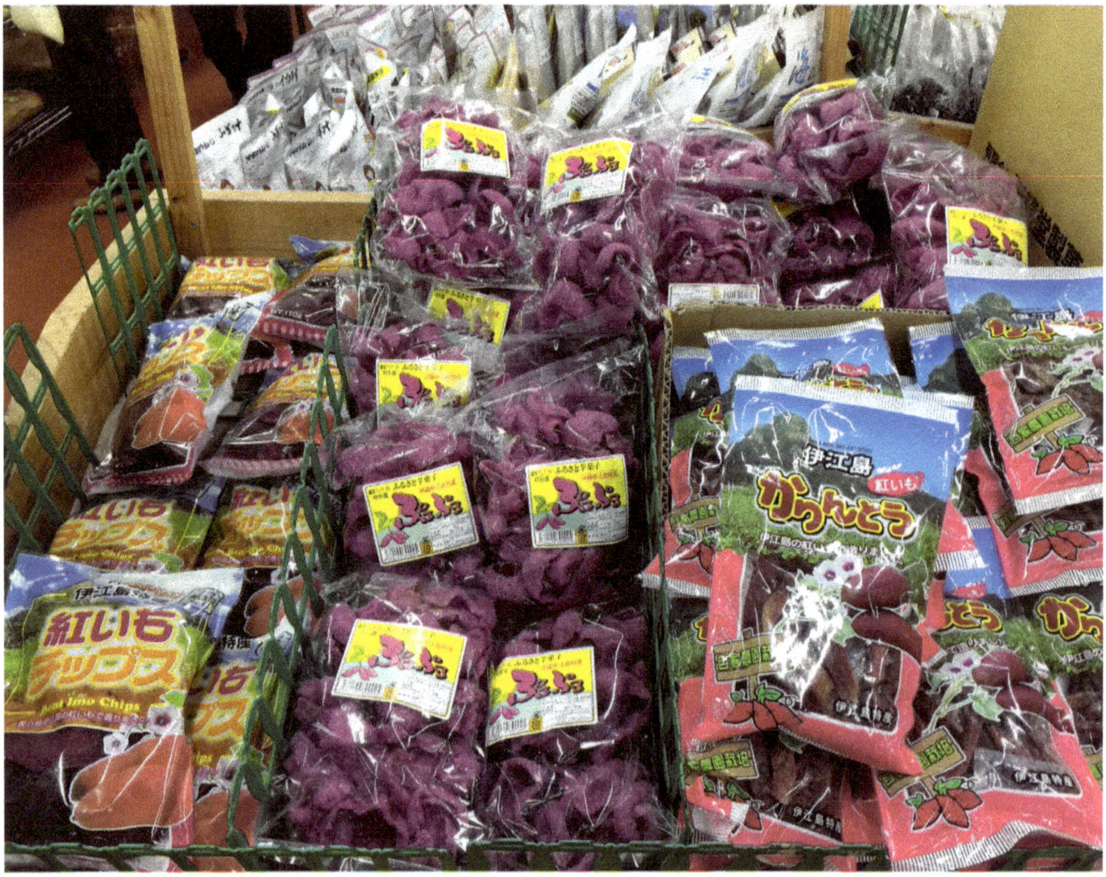

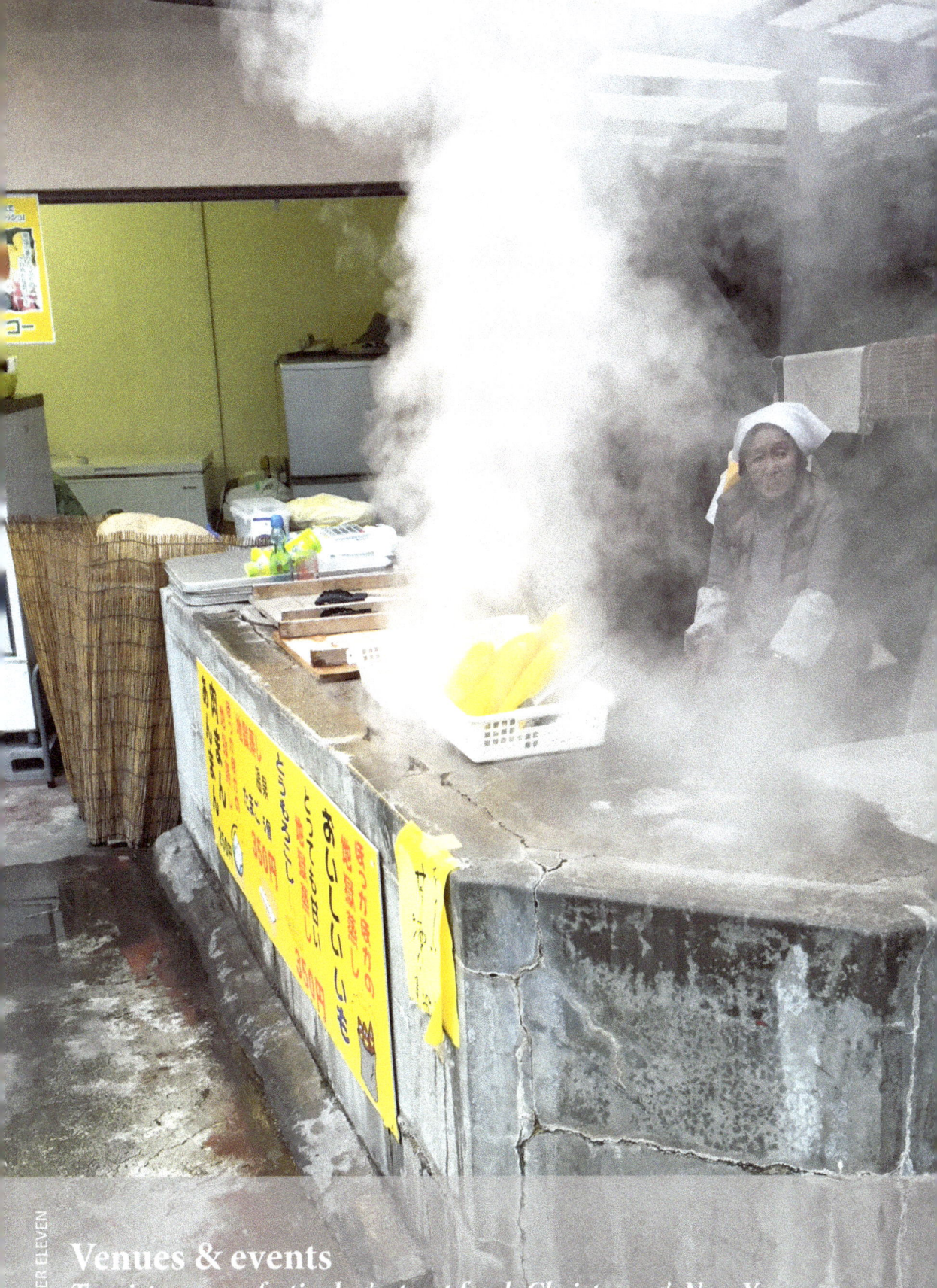

Venues & events
Tourist venues, festivals & street food, Christmas & New Year

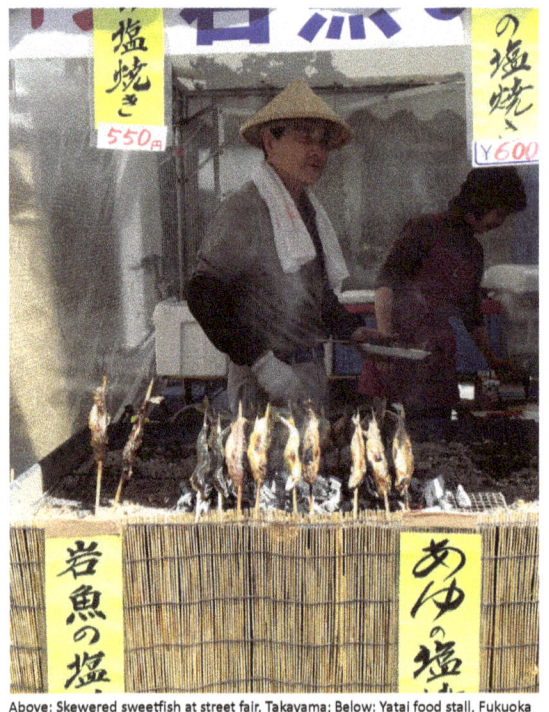
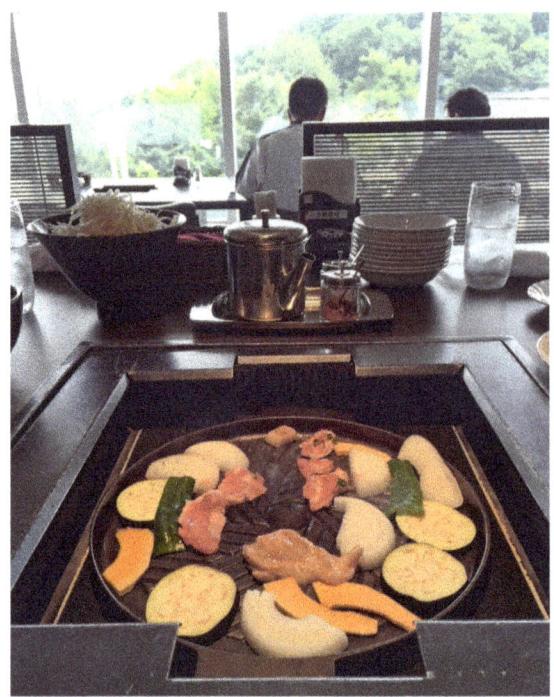

Above: Skewered sweetfish at street fair, Takayama; Below: Yatai food stall, Fukuoka   Above: Barbecue restaurant at Okurayama Ski Jump, Sapporo

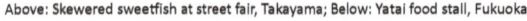

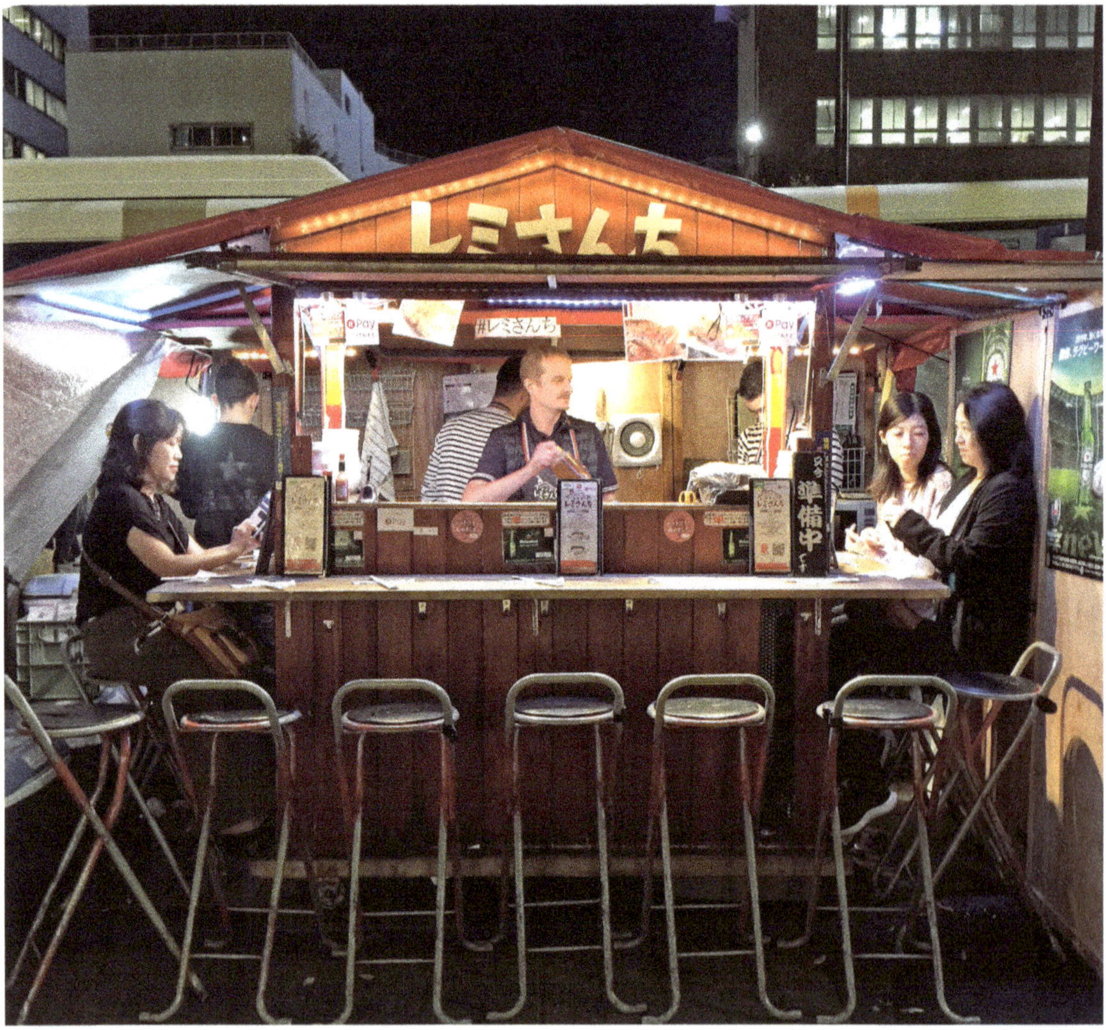

VENUES & EVENTS: Tourist venues, festivals & street food, Christmas & New Year

Tourist venues

Expect the unexpected in restaurants at tourist venues in Japan. Or rather, expect the usual! Unlike in Australia, where you normally pay inflated prices for meals at museums, art galleries, aquaria, botanic gardens and other tourist venues, in Japan the cost of eating at these places is similar to the cost at restaurants everywhere else. It's fair to say that in Japan you normally get what you pay for.

There were some venues that we visited several times because they were so good that we happily went back with different groups of friends. The first time we visited the Okurayama Ski Jump & Winter Sports Museum in Sapporo we bought some small snack foods and avoided the classy looking restaurant with the lovely view. The next time we decided to try the restaurant and found it to have an excellent barbecue menu featuring vegetables, chicken and/or lamb (Australian!), which we cooked on a hotplate at our own table. The food was great, the view was terrific and the price was very reasonable, so we went there later with a third group of friends.

We found that the same applied to most of the restaurants at tourist venues — such as the National Museum of Art in Fukuoka, the Hakone Open Air Sculpture Museum, the Sapporo Art Museum (delicious buffet with a special price for seniors), the Umitamago Aquarium in Beppu, and even at the airport in Fukuoka. So don't be nervous about eating in restaurants at venues.

Festivals & street food

We attended a number of different types of festivals, including the Hojoya festival in Fukuoka, the Naked Man festival in Okayama, the Sanja Matsuri festival in Tokyo, as well as several community fairs and a weekend food and drink festival in Takayama. At all these events most of the food wasn't gluten-free but we looked at each stall carefully and found suitable food — such as corn on the cob, barbecued octopus, salted yakitori, various sorts of potatoes (spirals, chips, whole, chopped up with mayonnaise), hard boiled eggs, tacos, sweetfish or tofu skewers and sushi, and sweet things like chocolate-coated bananas, ice creams and hot mochi (sweet rice balls).

Large flower festivals, sumo tournaments, markets, fish markets and beer festivals also have similar types of food available, though some will be local variations of the theme and foods may differ from season to season. Particularly nice on a cold winter's day are the skewered sweetfish (freshwater fish) or chicken skewers cooked vertically in beds of charcoal. Pounded rice sticks cooked over charcoal are also delicious, though you may have to ask for them not to be brushed with soy sauce (choose a miso option if available). Hot sweet potatoes are also good on a winter's day.

As with elsewhere around the world, most street food involves wheat products, so make sure you avoid okinomiyaki (cabbage pancakes), taiyaki (fish-shaped cakes filled with red beans), takoyaki (octopus dumplings), etc. One night in Fukuoka we found a range of gluten-free options at a French 'yatai' — a mobile street stall seating seven to eight people.

Christmas & New Year

In Japan Christmas is spent with friends, whereas New Year is the time spent with family before the start of a week-long holiday. At this time of year it can be difficult to get bookings and the transport is always crowded. Christmas Day is just like any other day, with the shops open and KFC on the menu (not an option for coeliacs!). If you go to any parties, you'll have to take your own gluten-free food, maybe some salted yakitori, sushi, sashimi or a chicken salad.

We were fortunate to be invited to spend New Year's Eve with the extended family of an Airbnb host. Everybody contributed to a communal meal, bringing either bought or homemade dishes that were laid out on a table for everyone to help themselves to. The food was varied and there were plenty of dishes that were gluten-free. As in Australia, the men and women tended to gravitate into separate groups, the children ran riot around the room, a lot of alcohol was consumed, and the TV was on until the final countdown to midnight. After which we walked to the local shrine for prayers.

Photo Page 49: Corn cooked in geothermal steam, Beppu

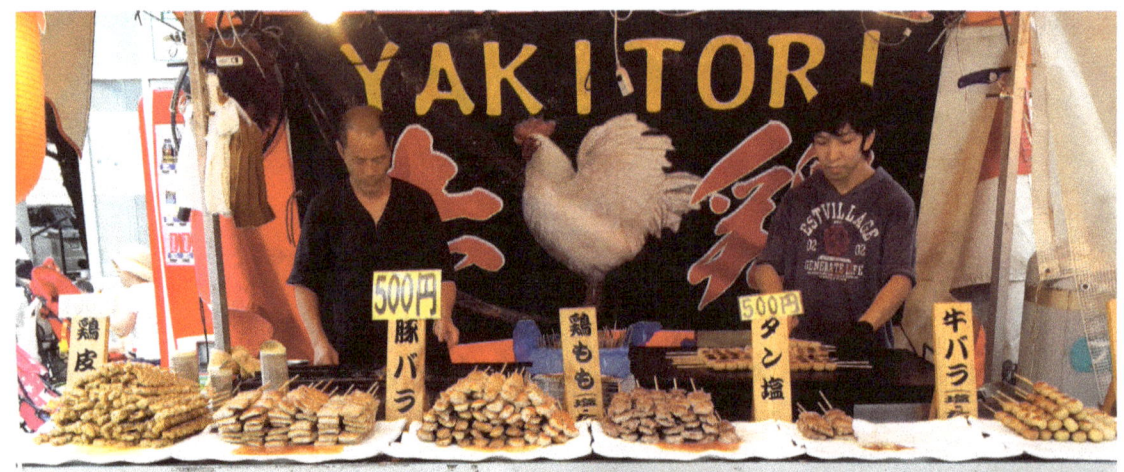
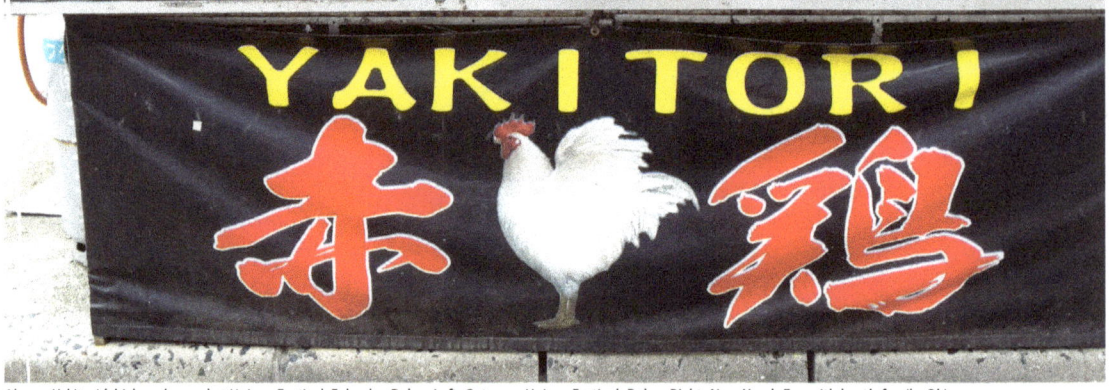

Above: Yakitori (chicken skewers) at Hojoya Festival, Fukuoka; Below Left: Octopus, Hojoya Festival; Below Right: New Year's Eve with host's family, Okinawa

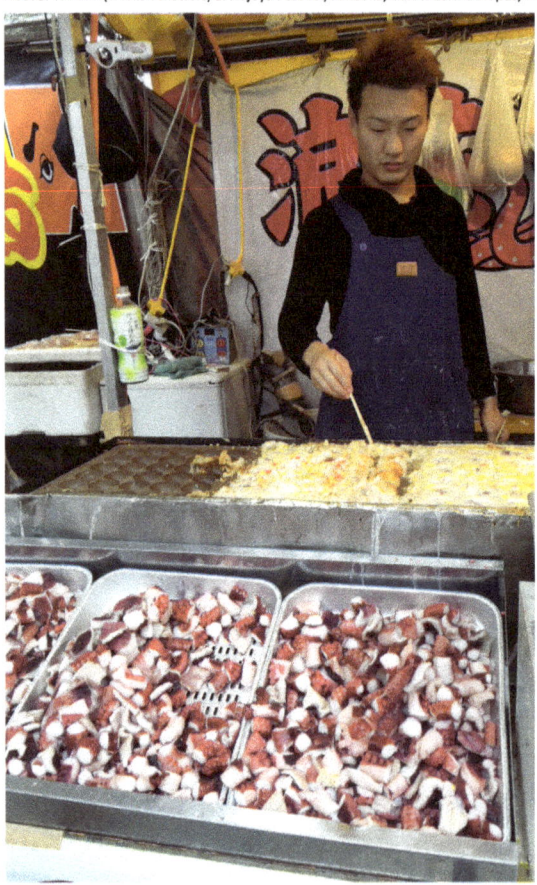
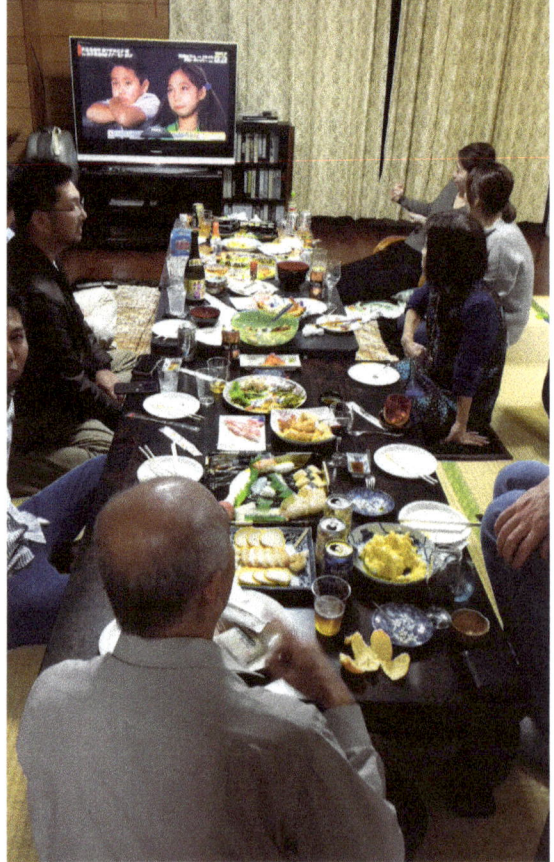

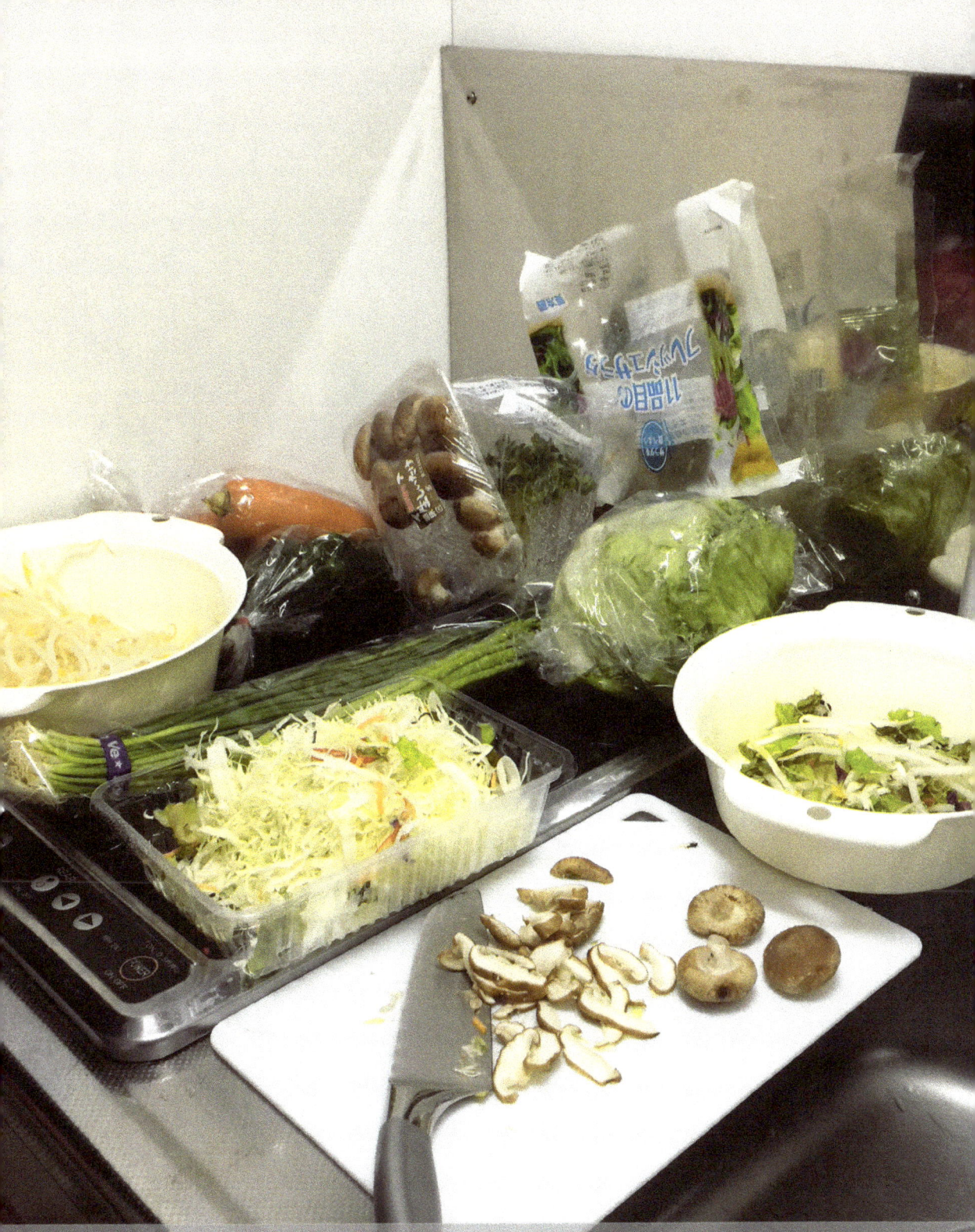

Cooking at home
Kitchen appliances, utensils, crockery & cutlery

CHAPTER TWELVE

53

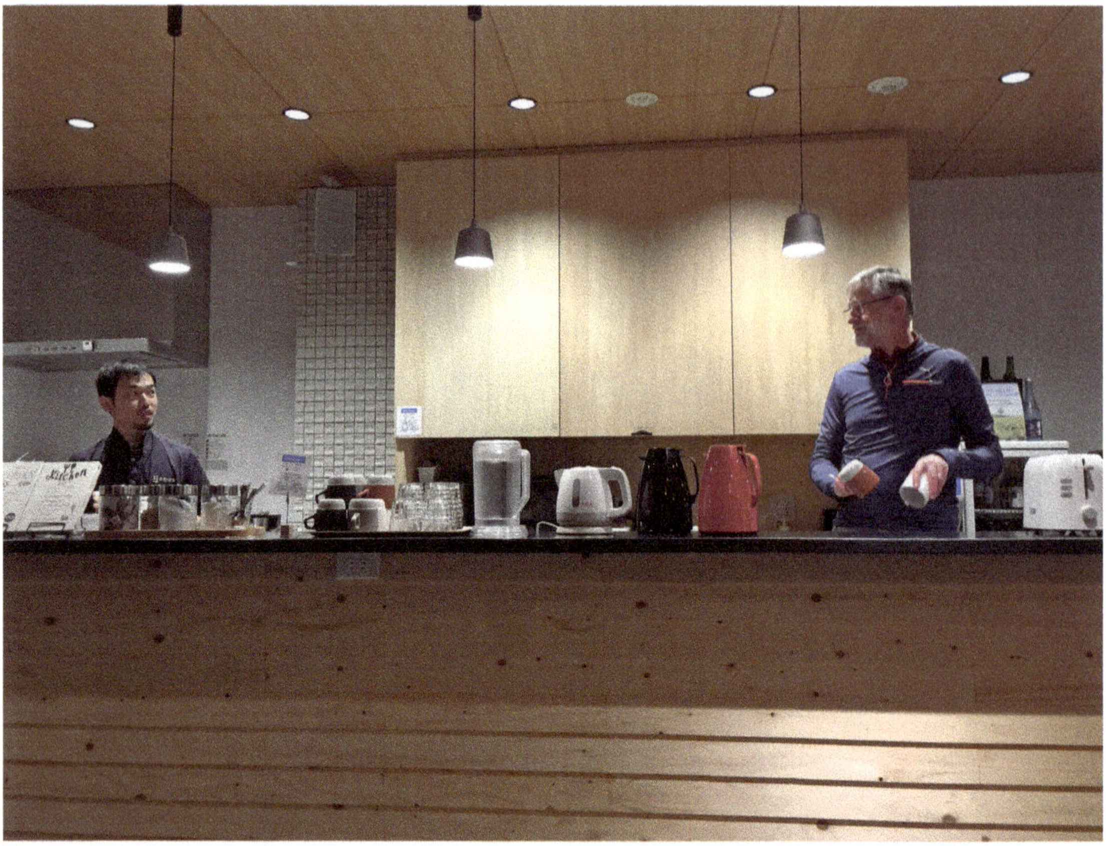

Above: Shared kitchen in Grids Hotel and Hostel in Sapporo; Below Left: Typical compact AirBnB kitchen; Below Right: Beautiful crockery in Airbnb, Kochi

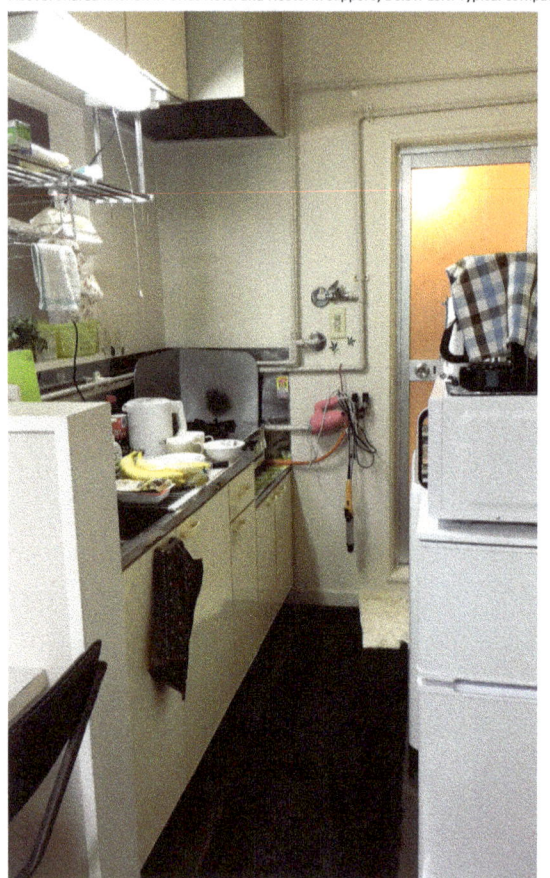
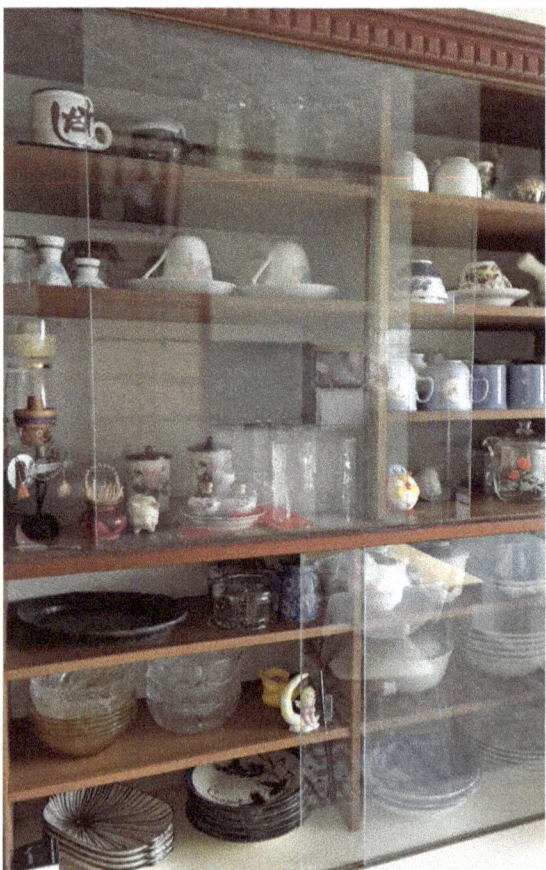

COOKING AT HOME: Kitchen appliances, utensils, crockery & cutlery

Kitchen appliances

Typically, as you'd expect, Japanese kitchens are quite small and compact. We stayed in a variety of Airbnbs, which gave us a good idea of what you'd expect in a basic Japanese kitchen — a cooktop (stovetop or portable single burner), which can be electric or gas, possibly induction and thus requiring special pans; a refrigerator (usually medium-sized, not as small as you'd find in a hotel); a microwave oven; an electric jug. Added extras might include a rice cooker, a toaster, and a proper oven. Occasionally we came across unusual appliances such as an electric dish dryer. The equipment in Airbnbs is usually fairly clean or easily cleaned — we rarely found anything too nasty apart from kitchen sink drains.

In Japan the authorities are very demanding with regard to waste disposal (although this varies from place to place). Because water is plentiful, the Japanese way of washing dishes is to use a sponge with detergent applied and wash under running hot water. Thus the plug doesn't get much use. If you take the plug out you'll find a fine mesh basket underneath that catches virtually any sized food scraps and prevents them from entering the waste system. Hopefully the Airbnb host has left a packet of these disposable mesh sieves somewhere in a cupboard, because they get mighty smelly and need to be emptied or disposed of regularly. There's a different sort of mesh to capture bathroom waste and these tend to become clogged with long black hair.

Be prepared to have to sort out your kitchen rubbish into at least three or four different bins, and to use the appropriate bags. There may be up to 14 different categories for recycling (e.g. paper/cardboard, PET bottles, glass, aluminium, etc.) as Japan has little room for landfill.

Utensils

The basic utensils that you should find in an Airbnb kitchen include a saucepan and a frying pan, as well as several implements such as an egg slice, large spoon (or cooking chopsticks), large and small knife, and a chopping board. If you're lucky there may be a range of pots and pans, but don't rely on it. We carried a saucepan of our own, as well as a sharp knife. You might or might not be provided with a colander, mixing bowl(s), vegetable peeler or other things you would normally use. If you can fit them in your luggage, these items can be picked up cheaply at a hundred-yen shop and carried around with you.

Crockery & cutlery

The same goes for crockery and cutlery. You might be provided with little more than a couple of flat plates and small bowls, a couple of glasses and cups, a knife and spoon or two and some chopsticks. So it's a good idea to carry a basic set of your own cutlery, as well as bowls and mug or two — again, these are cheap to buy and can be left at the accommodation or thrown away at the end of your stay.

But that's the worst case scenario! Most Airbnbs are well equipped with enough pots and pans, crockery and cutlery, and cooking gadgetry. You simply have to bear in mind that the expectation is that Airbnb customers in Japan are more likely to eat out or bring home ready-made meals from the supermarket than to go the trouble of cooking anything. Cooking is probably only an option for long-term travellers who might yearn for home-cooked meals and who stay at one accommodation for long enough to accumulate groceries — or those with special dietary requirements like coeliacs. Cooking your own meals in Japan probably isn't going to save you much money.

At the other end of the scale, we stayed in several Airbnbs that were incredibly well equipped. One place was a large house situated right next door to the host. We counted over 30 doorways connecting the vast number of rooms. It was quite possibly a place inherited from the host's parents as it had a lifetime's worth of beautiful crockery and cutlery — all of which we were welcome to use. Likewise, we stayed at several other Airbnbs that were immaculate and had beautiful locally produced glassware and crockery that we enjoyed using.

Photo Page 53: Cooking in apartment, Fukuoka

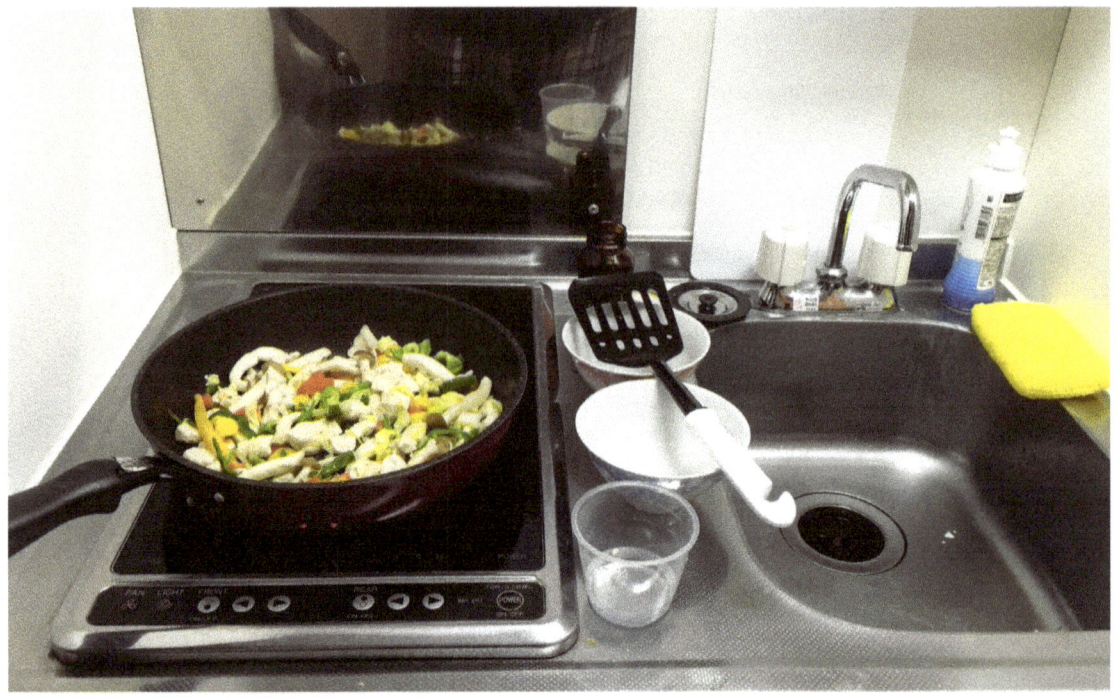

Above: Cooking in apartment, Fukuoka; Below: Well-equipped Airbnb kitchen, Sakaiminato

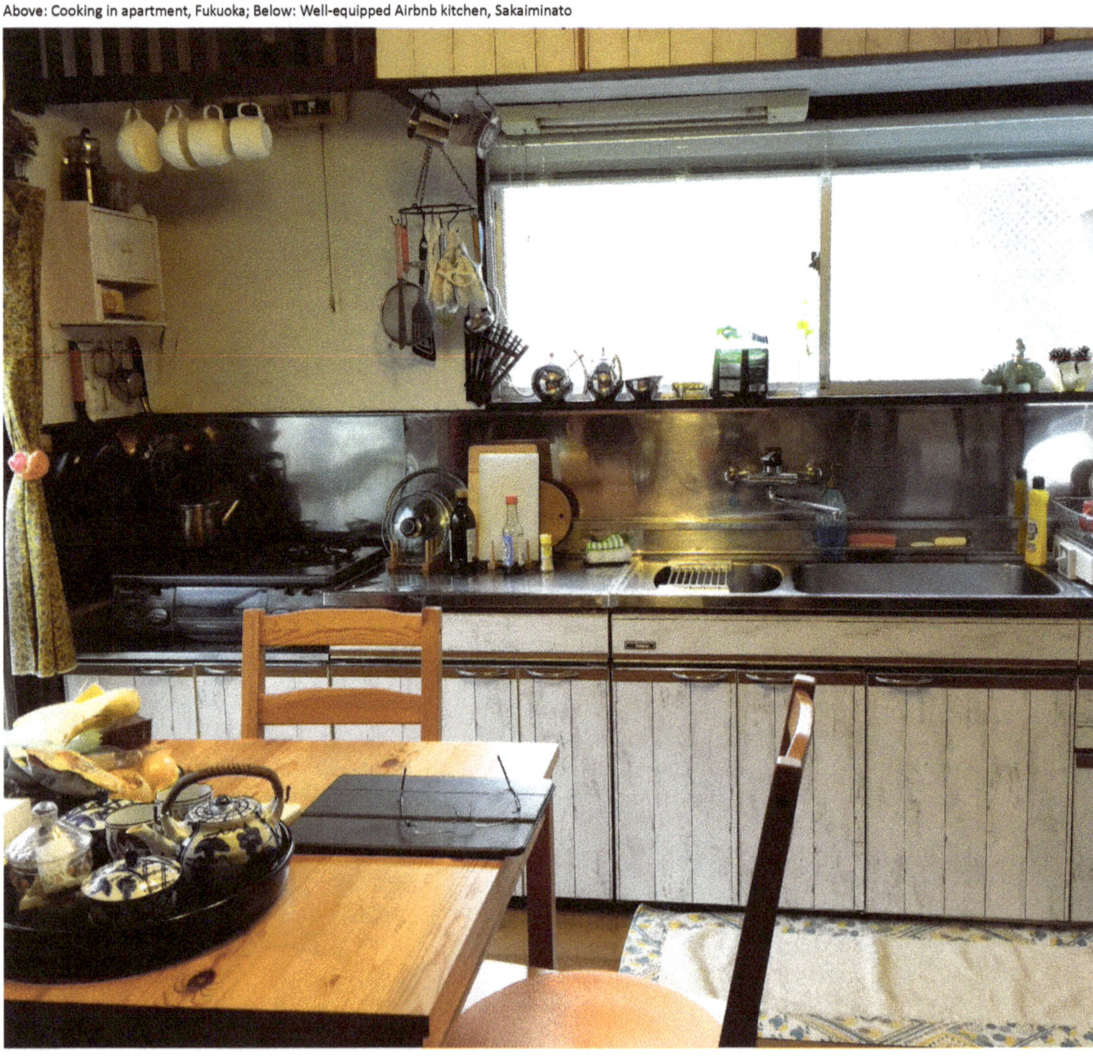

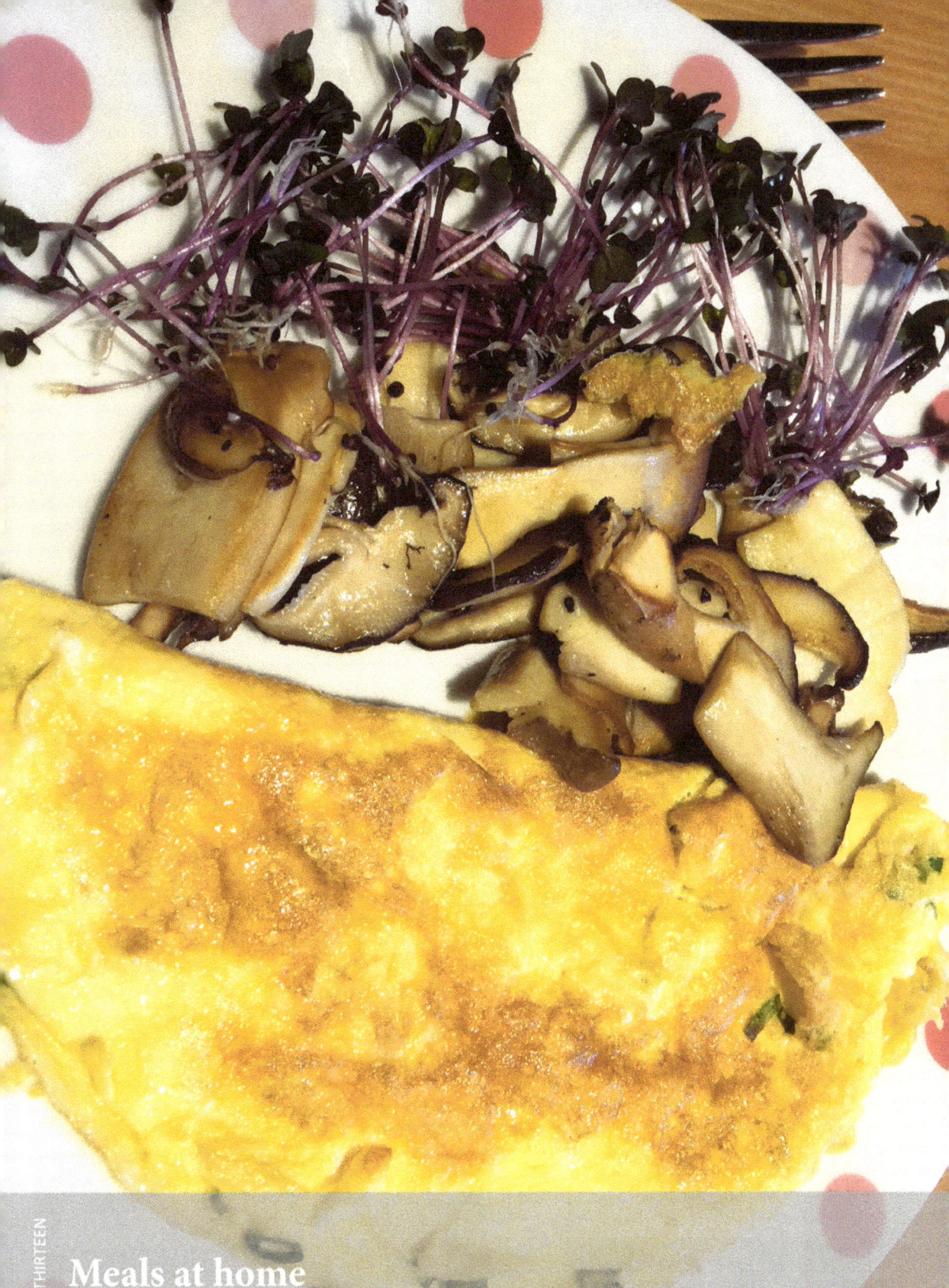

CHAPTER THIRTEEN

Meals at home
Breakfasts, lunches & dinners

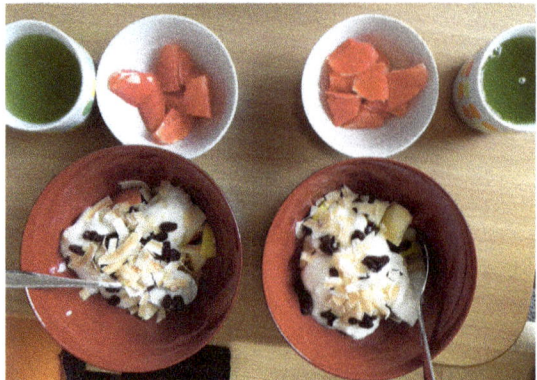
Above: Breakfast of yoghurt, sultanas and toasted coconut, blood oranges & matcha

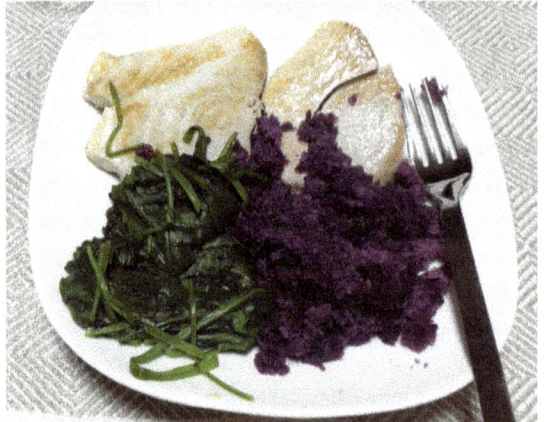
Below: Japanese breakfast at home, with fish, omelette, rice, pickles and miso soup

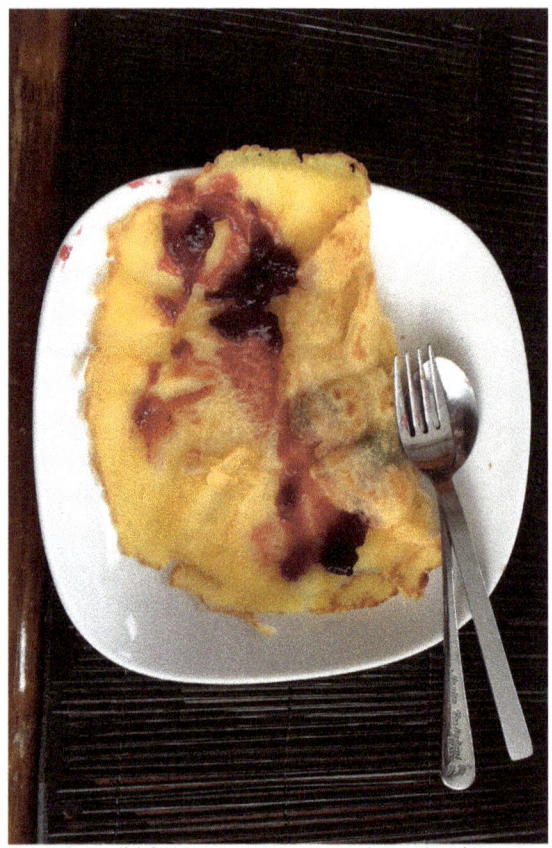
Above Left: Swordfish & Okinawan vegetables; Above Right: Pancake with jam

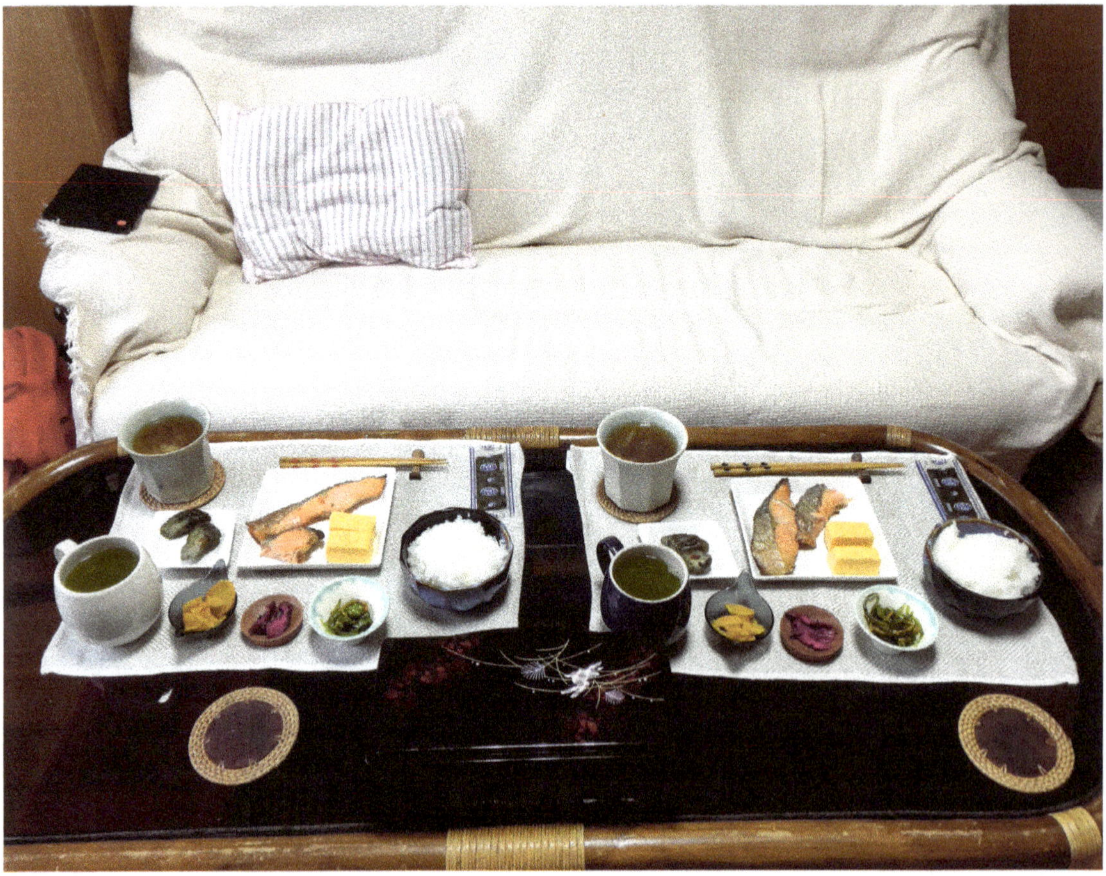

MEALS AT HOME: Breakfasts, lunches & dinners

Breakfasts

Sometimes Japanese accommodation, such as hotels and hostels, offer their guests a continental (or Western) breakfast. However, most of them have a delicious buffet breakfast that has a mixture of Japanese and Western (and sometimes Chinese) dishes. Once you've eaten at such buffets, it's easy to figure out what your favourite Japanese breakfasts are and then you can emulate them at home and put together your own breakfast feast — serve it as small amounts on individual plates (traditionally not matching) and serve with 'matcha' (instant green tea).

Lunches

Most of the time, when you're travelling around and away from your accommodation during the day, it's good to go to a restaurant for lunch then cook dinner at home after you've returned in the evening. Doing it this way around is a lot more economical, because there are lots of cheap lunch deals, whereas dinners tend to be a lot more expensive.

If you are heading home for lunch, the first option is to pick up a prepared meal from the supermarket when you get off the bus or train. But if you want to prepare something to eat, then a salad is a great idea. You'll find a plethora of vegetables and pickles either in the supermarket or, more cheaply, at a local fruit and vegetable shop. You'll find these shops in most neighbourhoods and the produce is always guaranteed to be fresh. There are many delicious varieties of vegetables. The range is much more extensive than found in Australia with many more colours available — so your salad will be colourful as well as attractive. For protein, add boiled eggs or some cooked salmon.

It's worth noting that many prepared meals at the supermarket are progressively marked down in price from the early evening on. So you might pick up a bargain either for dinner or to keep for the next day's lunch. But later at night you might find that your favourites have all been sold!

Dinners

Dinners are easy to prepare, especially if you have your own gluten-free soy sauce to use in stir fries (serve with instant rice) and gluten-free flour to use in other dishes. You can prepare some of the meals that you can't sample in restaurants.

Breakfast suggestions
- Japanese style: salmon, omelette, rice, miso soup, pickles, fruit, salad, yoghurt, tofu & matcha
- Fresh bananas/figs/strawberries, yoghurt, sultanas & shredded coconut
- Left-over rice with fruit, sultanas & shredded coconut
- Omelette with mushrooms & tomatoes
- GF pancakes with jam or fruit and yoghurt

Lunch suggestions
- Meal/snack from convenience store or supermarket e.g. sushi, sashimi, onigiri
- Salad with mushrooms, lettuce, onion, sprouts, tomatoes, carrots, capsicums & hard boiled eggs or cooked salmon

Dinner suggestions
- 'Oyakodon' (literally 'parent and child' — egg and chicken served on rice)
- 'Okinomiyaki' (cabbage pancake incorporating vegetables or meat of your choice and made with gluten-free flour)
- 'Karaage' chicken (chicken coated with gluten-free flour and deep fried)
- GF noodles or spaghetti with tomato and meat sauce or clams
- Stir fried vegetables, chicken, tofu, prawns or beef
- Fried rice or paella
- Tacos (shells from Kaldi Coffee Farm or some supermarkets) or taco rice (taco filling on top of rice)
- Seaweed salad with fish, chicken or other meat
- Rice paper rolls with shredded vegetables and/or prawns

Photo Page 57: Omelette and mushrooms with spicy micro-greens

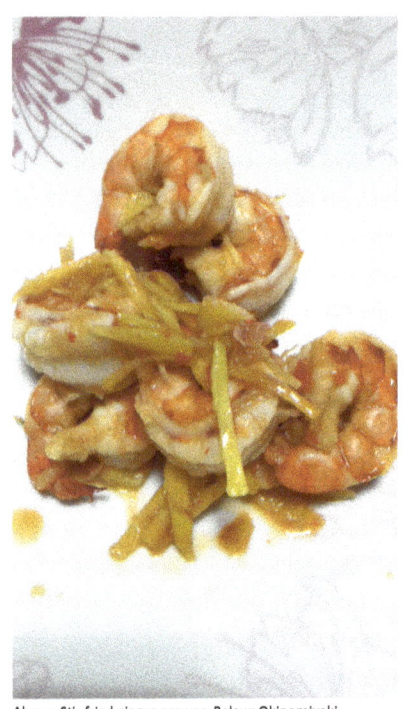
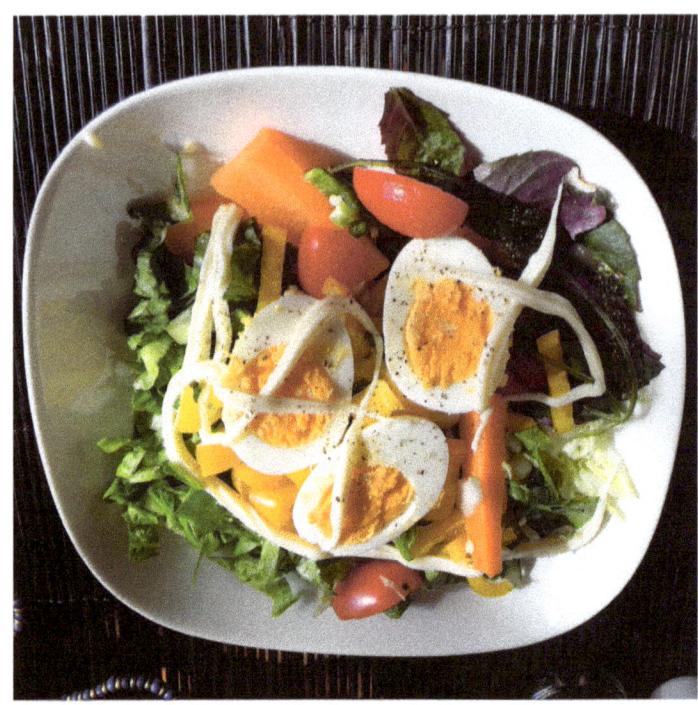

Above: Stir fried ginger prawns; Below: Okinomiyaki   Above: Salad lunch with hard boiled eggs; Below: Rice paper rolls with sweet chilli sauce

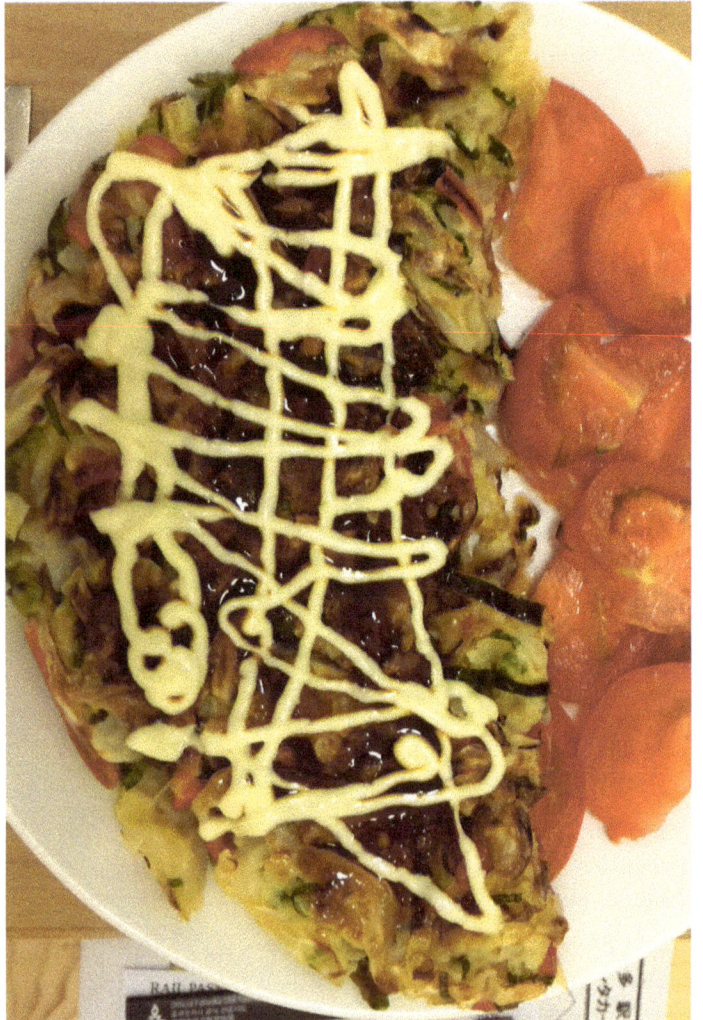
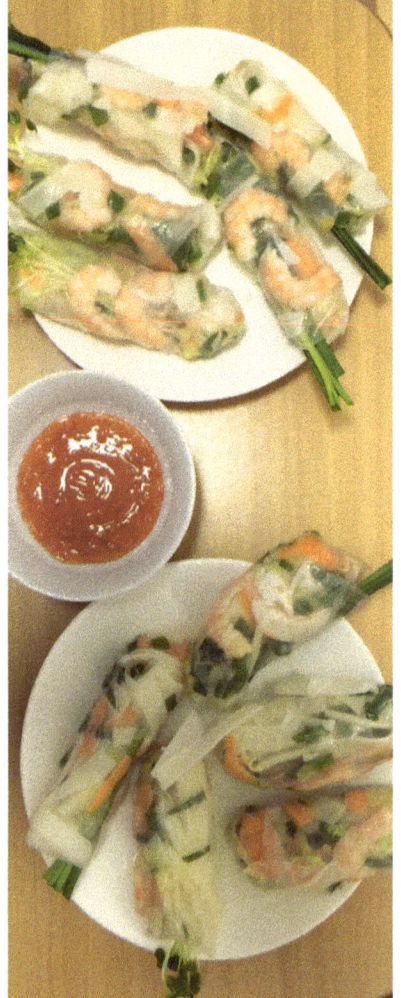

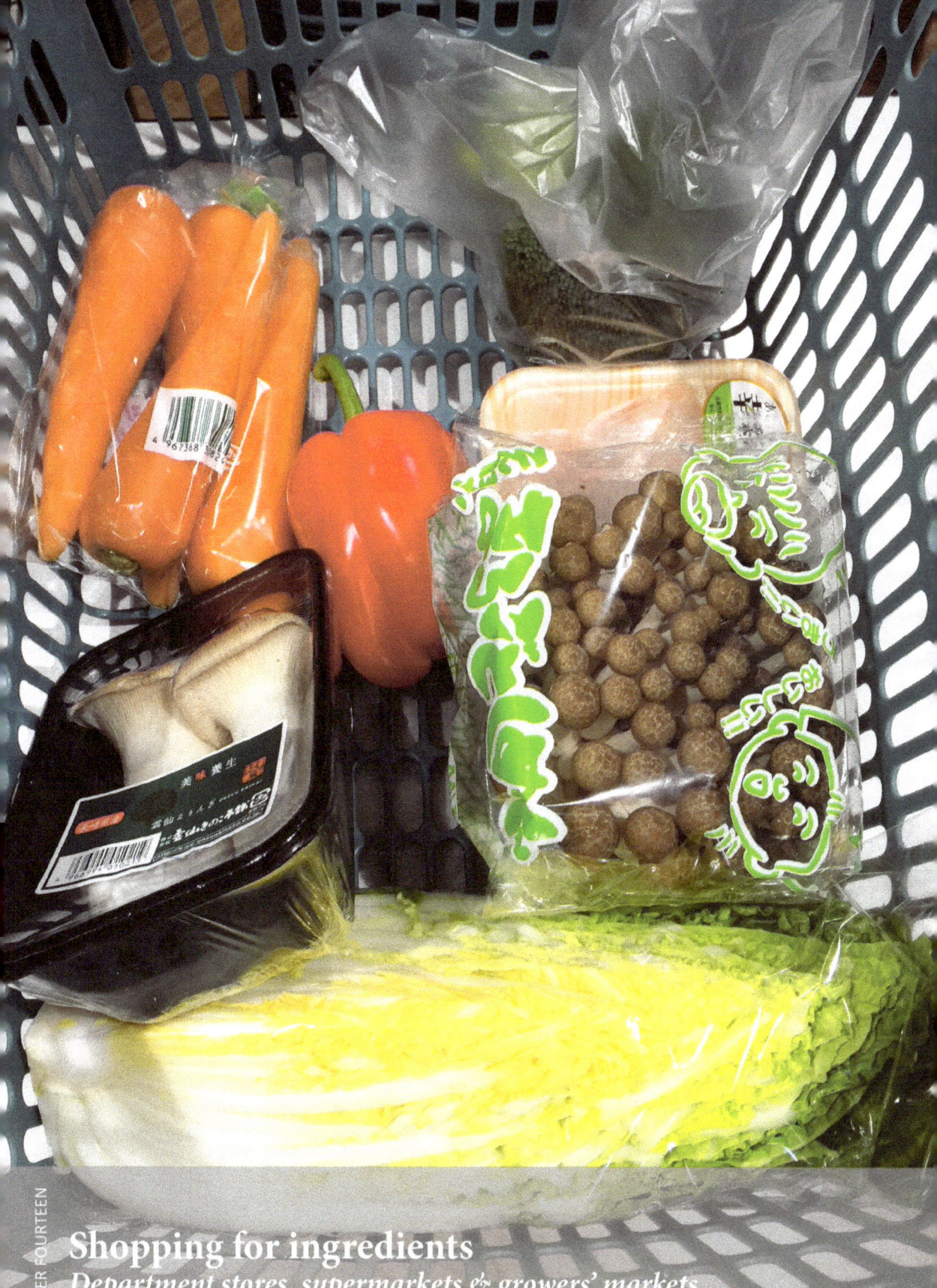

Shopping for ingredients
Department stores, supermarkets & growers' markets

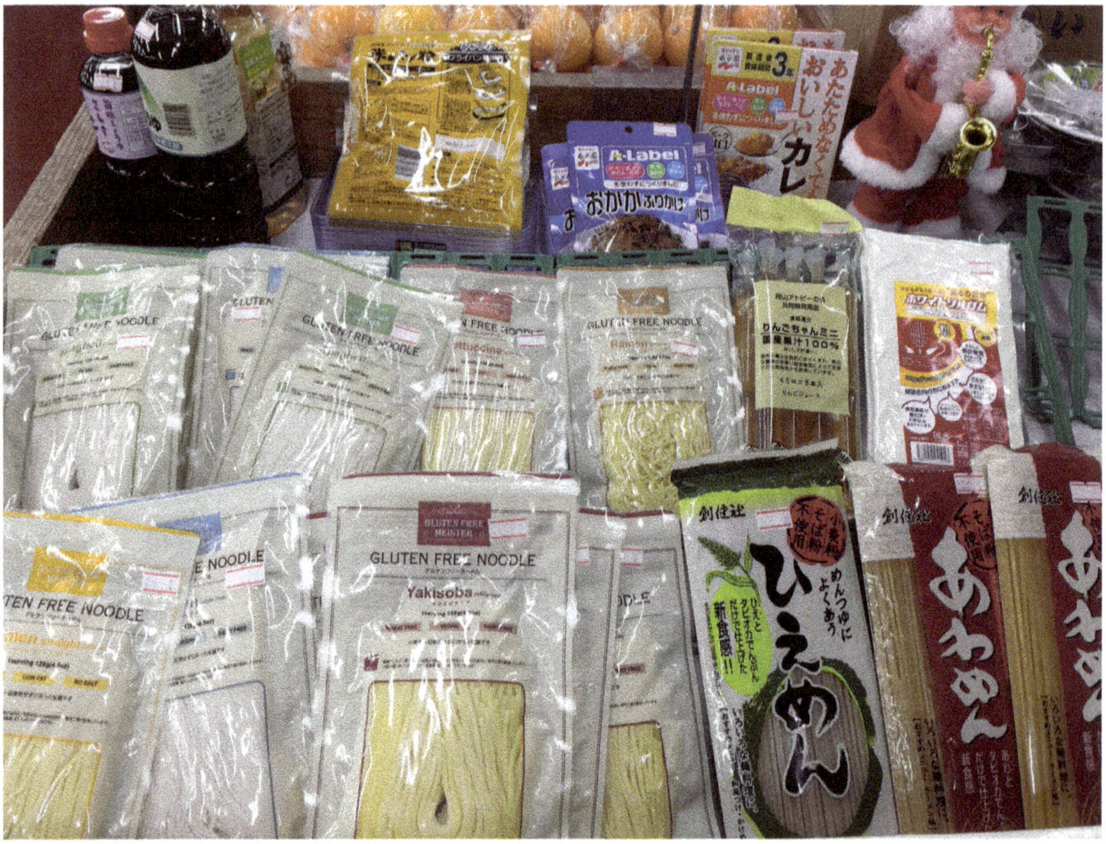

Above: Gluten-free products in Growers' Market, Itoman, Okinawa; Below: Egg section of supermarket, Tokyo

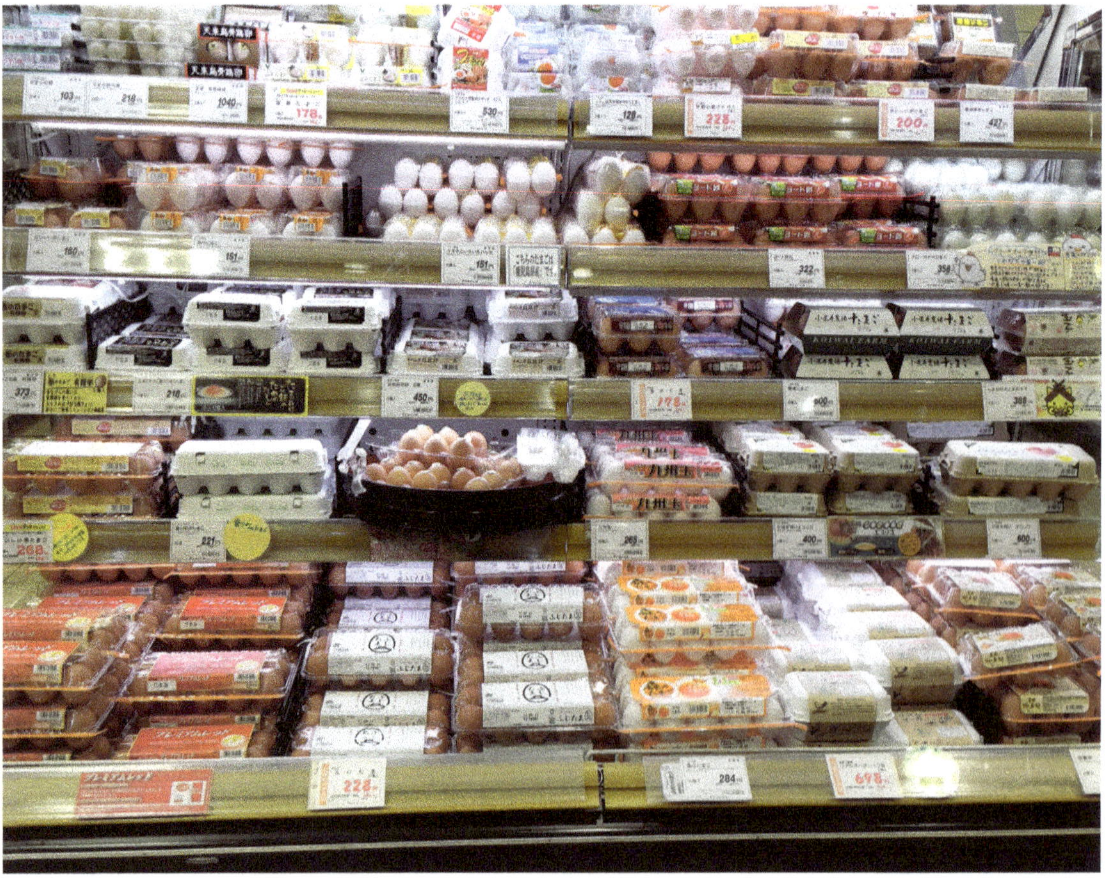

SHOPPING FOR INGREDIENTS: Department stores, supermarkets & growers' markets

Department stores

The food section of major department stores can usually be found on the ground or basement floors. It's certainly worth a look at the wonderful array of very expensive produce, often laid out in lavish displays. High-end department stores are, however, a good source of hard-to-find specialty products, such as different types of flour, or even tamari or gluten-free soy sauce. Apart from Okinawa, department stores were the only places in which we found gluten-free soy sauce (at a price, but they did wrap the bottles in bubble wrap!). It's best to do a bit of research so that you can recognise the packaging on the shelf.

Supermarkets

Supermarkets are the best place to buy your groceries as they usually stock everything from fruit and vegetables, to dairy, eggs, meat, packaged goods, drinks, including alcohol, and ready-made meals. They will have a good range of short-grained rice, including instant rice that you can microwave. They also often have a good bakery section, but virtually the only gluten-free products in it will be some mochi (sweet rice balls). Some supermarkets in Kyushu and Okinawa have a small section of gluten-free products — flour, pancake mix, noodles. The main gluten-free products you can be sure of finding in most large Japanese supermarkets are Soyjoy bars, fruit and vegetables, eggs, cheese, dairy, fish, chicken, red meat, tea, coffee, soft drinks, juices, wine, sake, spirits and nuts.

It might be difficult to find anything decent that is gluten-free in small rural supermarkets. On occasions when we were trekking and had to buy ahead for a picnic lunch, we could really only find a few things like strawberries, bananas, mandarins (mikans), chocolate, fish patties, nuts, and cheese in the smaller ones. If you're lucky, these small supermarkets may have the odd takeaway meal or onigiri (savoury rice balls). So, my advice would be to always keep a spare Soyjoy bar or two in your backpack.

Some supermarkets provide small ice packs for transporting cold foods home. They may be given to you at the checkout or you may have to look around in the packing area. Some supermarkets have an ice machine (free), or even a dry ice machine (which requires a token). Supermarkets usually take credit cards, although cash is more commonly used. The cash is counted by a machine that issues a receipt and dispenses the change.

Kaldi Coffee Farm mini-supermarkets are useful if you're homesick for foods from other countries, and they stock some useful gluten-free products — for example, Vietnamese rice paper roll wrappers, Malaysian toasted coconut, Mexican tacos and taco sauce.

Growers' markets

In both department stores and supermarkets, you need to look at labels and be able to recognise the characters for wheat especially, but also barley, rye and oats (see Introduction). The ingredients are usually listed in the main part of the label, whereas information on traces or other products processed in the same factory will be lower down. For many coeliacs, trace amounts won't present a problem, whereas for others it might. If you recognise the wheat character, scanning the label with Google Translate will help give an idea of whether there is gluten in the product itself or only a trace element from the factory.

Growers' markets are an excellent source of fresh produce, as are fish markets, supermarkets and specialty places that produce only one product, such as tofu shops. For the most part the food in these outlets is simple and the ingredients are easy to recognise. The grower's market in Itoman in Okinawa was perhaps the best source of gluten-free products that we came across in the whole of Japan. The products were also labelled in English! And that particular growers' market had the best range of fresh healthy fruit, vegetables and snack foods. The seafood market next door stocked an interesting range of fresh and cooked produce. So we could do our shopping and also enjoy a nice lunch. If you're walking around in the countryside, look out for small strange-looking buildings as they may house a rice-polishing machine, or an egg-vending machine!

Photo Page 61: Shopping in supermarket, Ohashi, Fukuoka

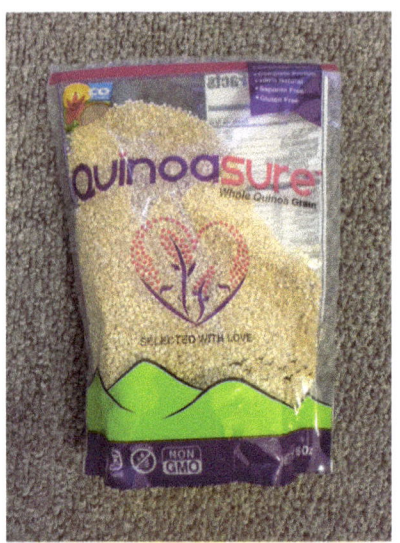
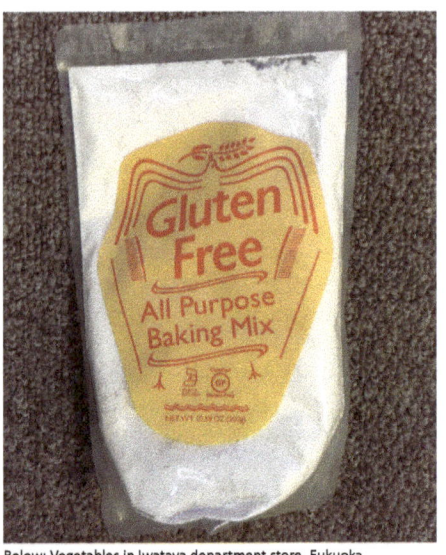
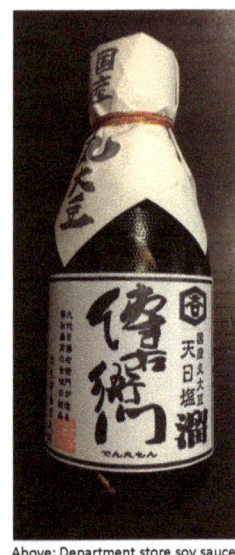

Above Left & Centre: Quinoa & flour, supermarket, Fukuoka   Below: Vegetables in Iwataya department store, Fukuoka   Above: Department store soy sauce

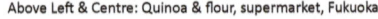

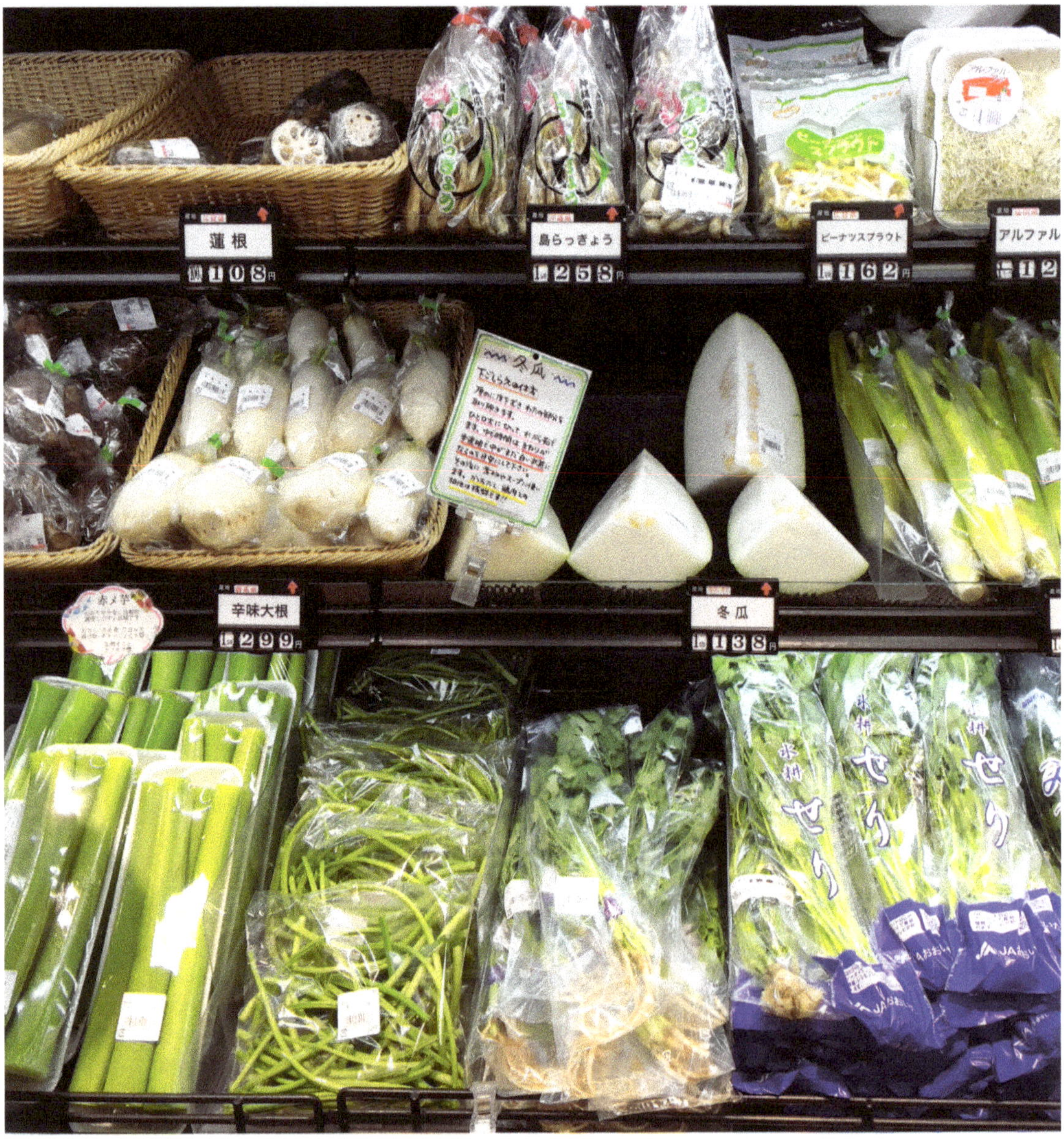

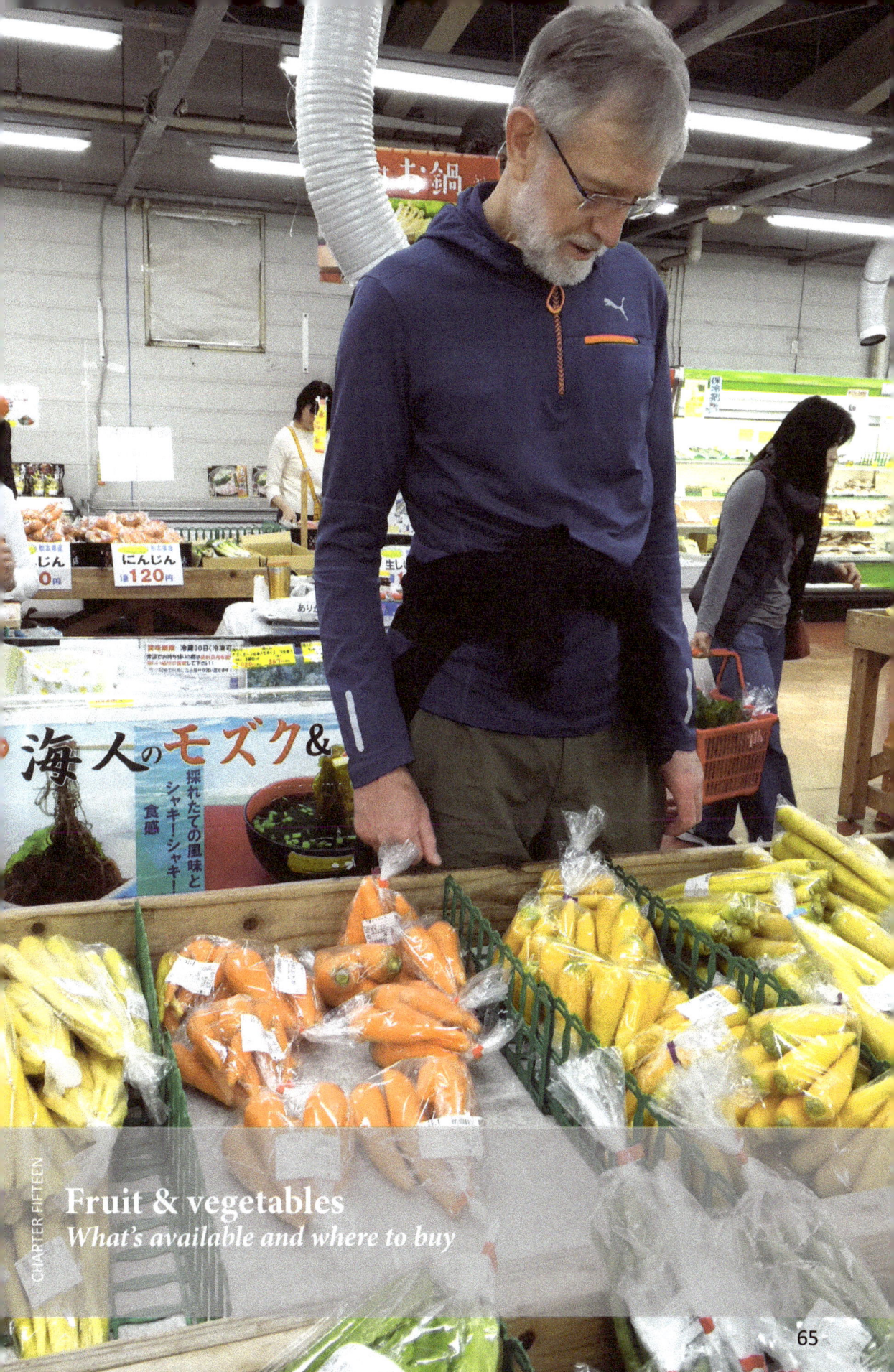

Fruit & vegetables
What's available and where to buy

CHAPTER FIFTEEN

65

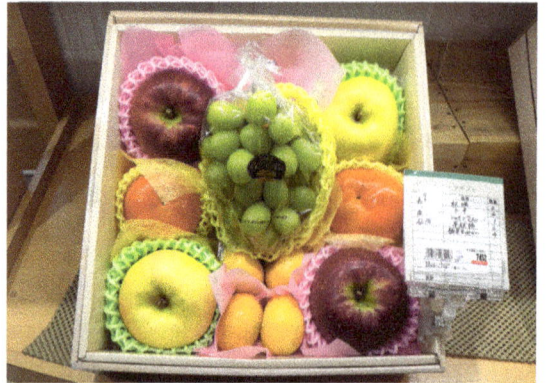
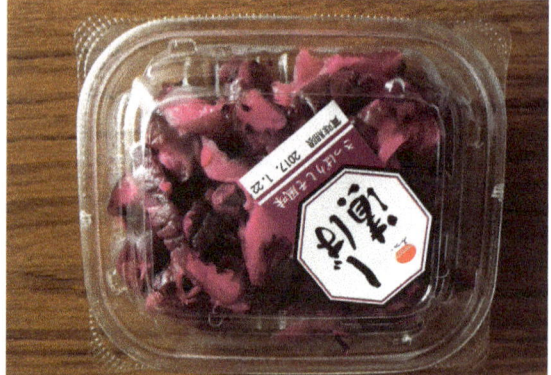

Above: $100 fruit basket in Iwataya Department Store, Fukuoka

Above: Pickled eggplant from supermarket, Okinawa

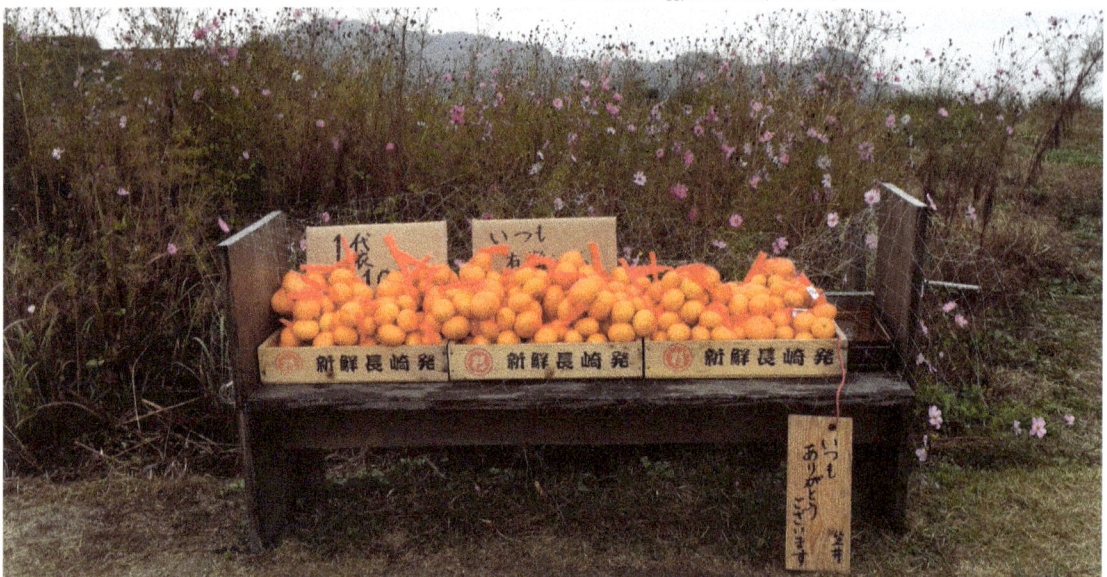

Above: Nagasaki mekans (mandarins) for sale, on Teshima Island; Below: Mushrooms in supermarket, Ohashi, Fukuoka

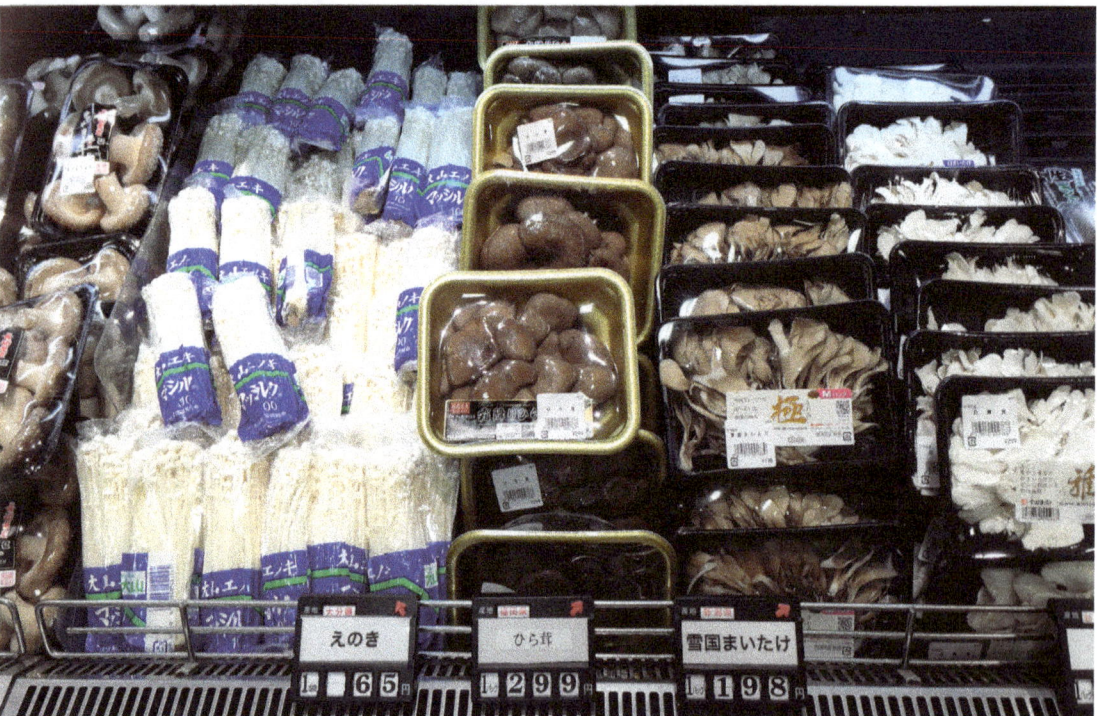

FRUIT & VEGETABLES — What's available & where to buy

Fruit

In Japan, fruit is usually of very high quality, wherever you buy it. In large department stores, where each item is as close to perfect as possible and carefully wrapped accordingly, fruit can be very expensive — e.g. cherries for $100 a box, apples for $10 each, a small bunch of grapes $60 or more, and musk melons for $150 or more each (displayed in their own special boxes in climate-controlled cabinets). But don't be dismayed. If you really want to buy things in a department store, you'll find some more reasonably priced and not-so-perfect produce in the same store and too not far away. However, the cheapest places to buy fruit (and vegetables) are supermarkets and green grocers.

Kyushu is known as the fruit bowl of Japan, with a wide range of produce that varies with the season. Summer fruits include cherries, peaches, melons, blueberries and grapes. In autumn there are chestnuts, pears, apples and mikan (mandarins) — the latter continuing in winter, at which time strawberries and kiwi fruit come into season. Not only can you buy these fruits in stores, but many orchards are open for picking excursions, where you pay by the hour to eat as many as you like. Much of Japanese fruit is grown in greenhouses, or in the open but covered with netting, or individual fruits are 'bagged'. The fruit seasons become progressively later as you head north, with the cherry and plum season extending through to summer in Hokkaido. In the very south of Japan, in subtropical Okinawa, bananas, mangoes, passionfruit and pineapples are abundant.

There's an incredible range of citrus available in Japan, especially in Shikoku. We found just about every type of citrus represented at the Kochi markets and along the 'Orange Train' railway route on the west coast, where citrus are celebrated with plantings at every station along the way. The large citrus called 'bankan' is even sometimes used as a gimmick, floating in local onsens in the area. The most common citrus in Japan is the mikan (mandarin) whereas the yuzu has the most interesting flavour and is fast becoming popular world-wide.

Vegetables

Vegetables in Japan tend to be cheaper than fruit. The range of vegetables (and salads) available in local supermarkets and suburban green grocers (a cheaper option) is mind-blowing. Like fruit, everything is fresh because of the rapid turnover and the Japanese insistence on quality. Tomatoes, for example, not only come in a large variety of sizes and colours but they also have incredible flavour. There's a huge range of pickles, sprouts and 'micro-greens' — from fresh bean sprouts to delicate peppery green and purple shoots — to add to salads.

But the 'vegetable' with the most amazing range of delicious varieties of all is the not-so-humble mushroom. Sometimes you'll come across whole display counters filled with ten, twenty or more different types of mushroom — from the dainty white enokitake with small heads and long stems, to the many bunched types of mushrooms, to the delicious and most popular shitake mushrooms (cultivated on rows of dead logs in rural areas) and the large meaty varieties of various colours. A selection of three of four different types of mushrooms fried up together in butter goes well with any salad, omelette or meat dish.

Sweet potatoes are popular in Japan. While you can only buy the beni-imo, or purple fleshed variety, in Okinawa, yellow fleshed sweet potatoes are more common elsewhere. Look for these hot treats in supermarkets, where they are to be found resting on hot coals in special cabinets.

Apart from the very healthy purple fleshed beni-imo, Okinawa boasts many other interesting and healthy vegetables. Bitter melons are popular here and in the south of Japan generally, but you'll also find yellow and purple varieties of carrots, and delicious green and purple leafy vegetables — which can be cooked like spinach. The growers' market we shopped at in Itoman in Okinawa also occasionally sold fresh wakame seaweed, which was delicious with finely sliced white onion, fresh tofu and gluten-free soy sauce. Blocks of tofu sold in supermarkets in Okinawa are so fresh that they are sometimes still warm.

Photo Page 65: Growers' market, Itoman, Okinawa

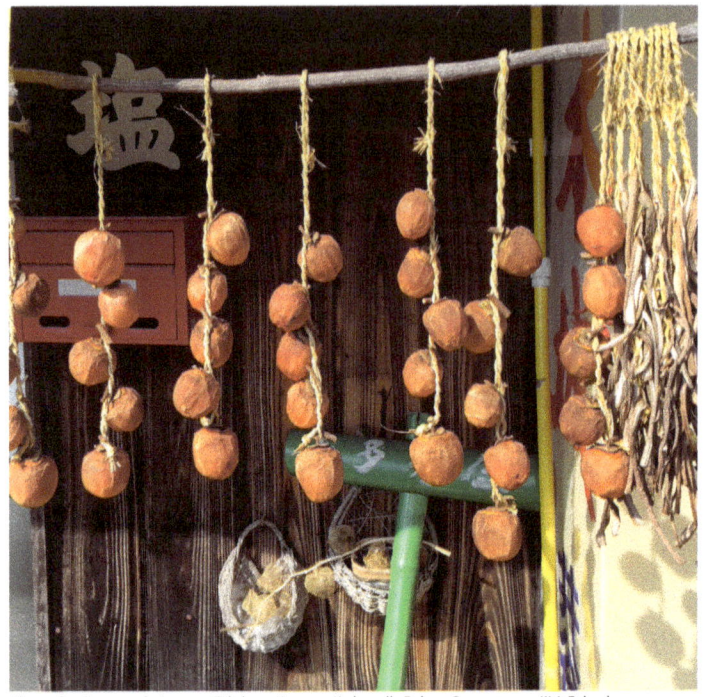
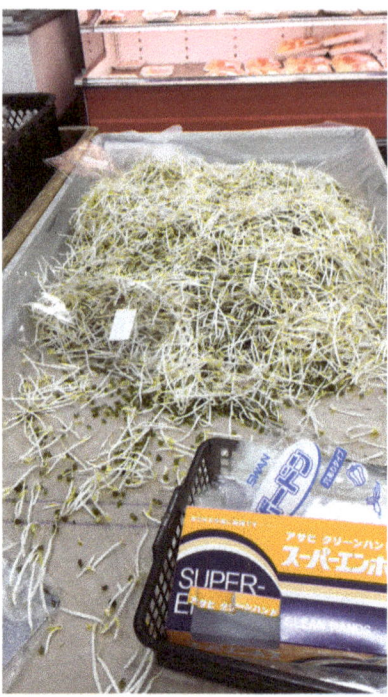

Above: Persimmons drying near Takahara, Kumano-Kodo walk; Below: Green grocer, Ijiri, Fukuoka　　Above: Bean sprouts at Growers' Market, Itoman, Okinawa

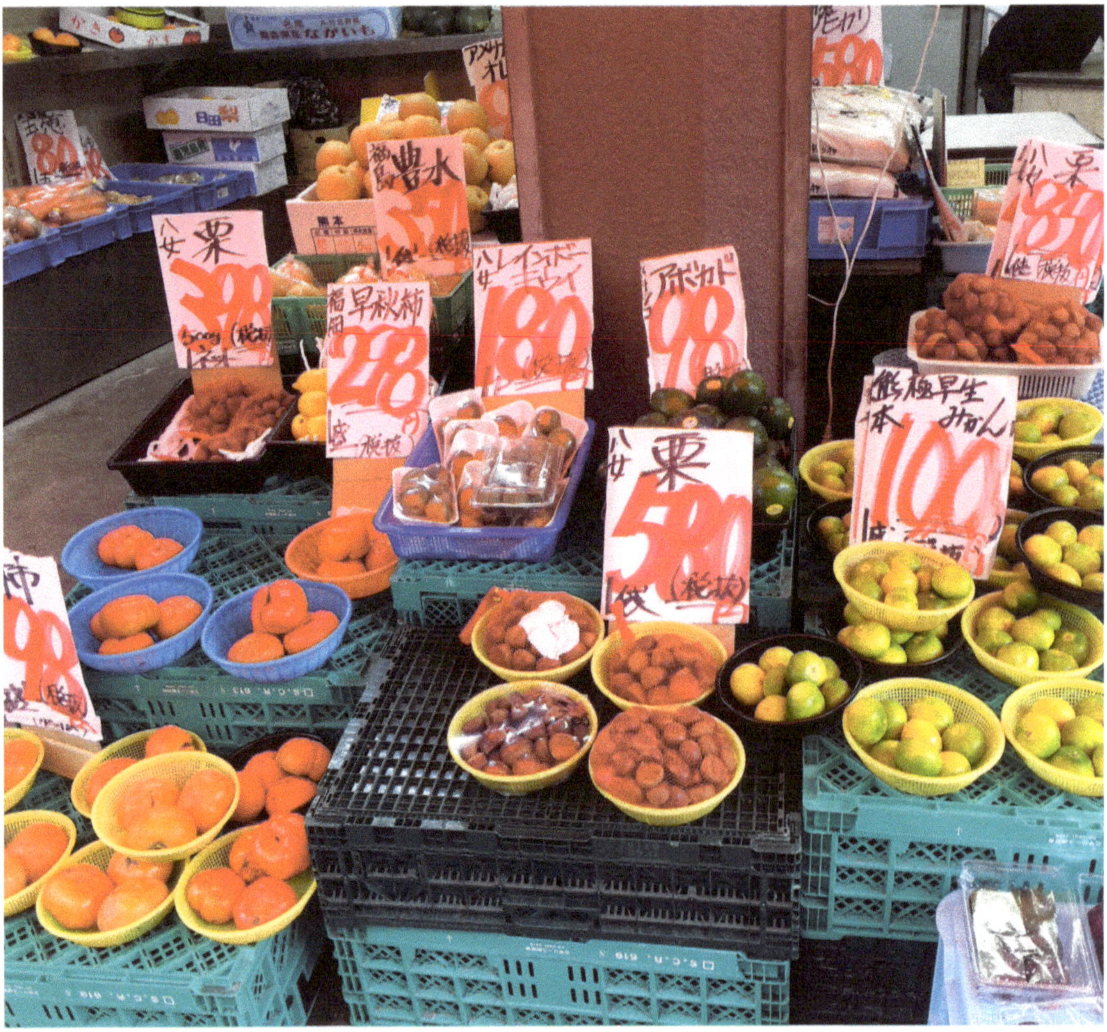

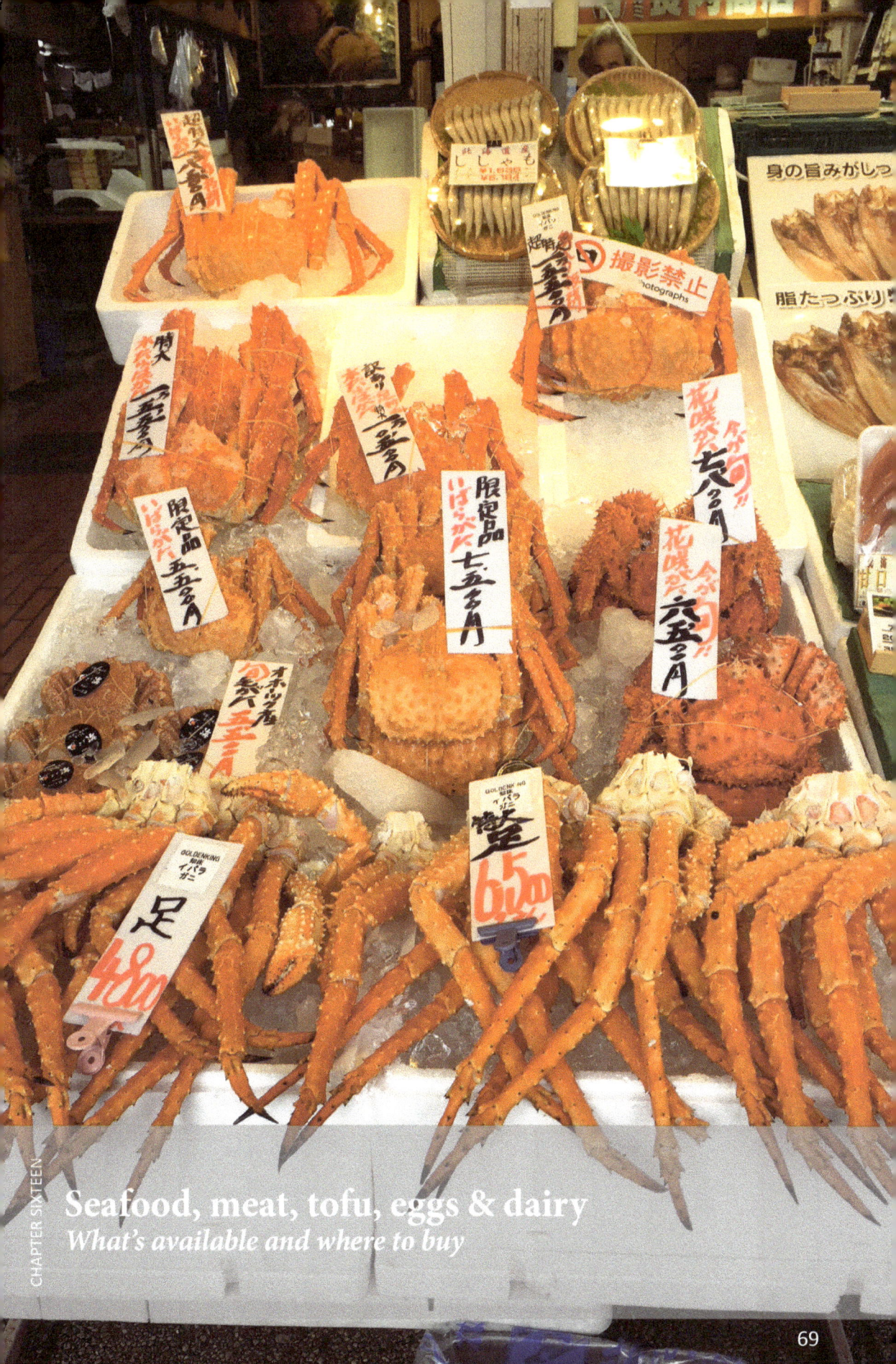

Seafood, meat, tofu, eggs & dairy
What's available and where to buy

CHAPTER SIXTEEN

69

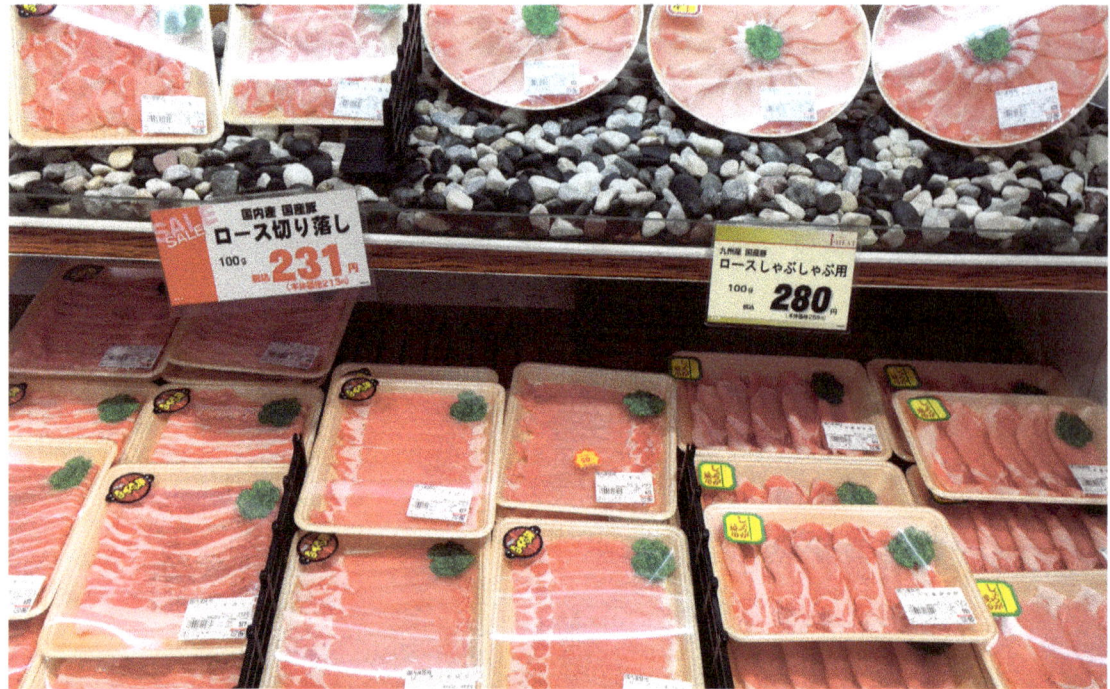

Above: Meat section of department store, Fukuoka; Below: Yakitori in supermarket, Kyoto — only the salted yakitori are gluten-free

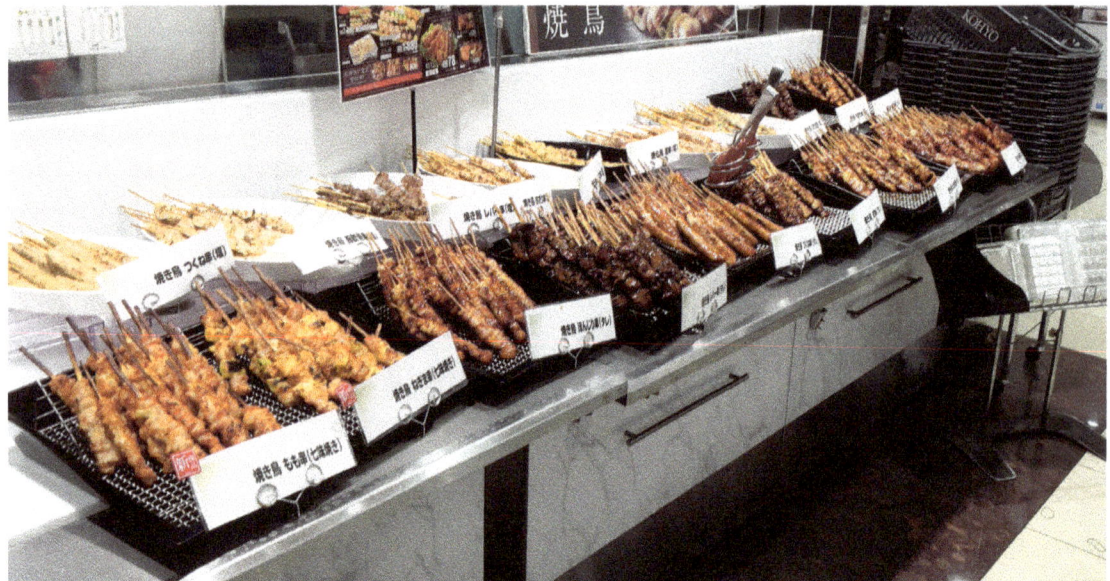

Below Left: Fish patties are usually gluten-free, supermarket, Tokyo; Below Right: Fresh tofu, Itoman, Okinawa

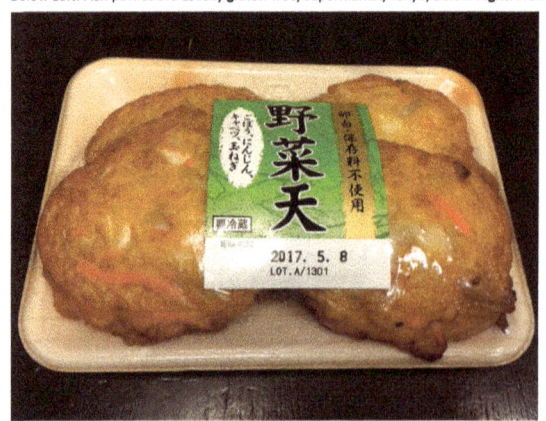
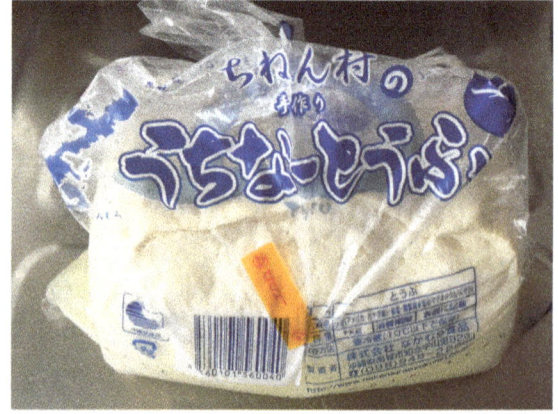

SEAFOOD, MEAT, TOFU, EGGS & DAIRY: What's available & where to buy

Seafood

Japan is well known for its excellent range of fresh seafood. Indeed, it would seem that all parts of fish, molluscs and other seafood are used, apart from the shells. We came across some very interesting bits and pieces that were very difficult to get our heads around eating — and also some that were worth trying but not very palatable. Some of the most interesting seafood we encounterd and actually ate were sliced octopus heads, octopus eggs, whelks, flying fish and blowfish. The tunicates and sea cucumbers we saw didn't seem very appealing and the abalone were far too expensive.

Fresh fish, cooked fish, pieces of fish (even heads), fish sashimi, fish sushi, fish patties, and so on, are to be found in most supermarkets. There are also specialised fish shops, as well as seafood markets. Of course, most fish in restaurants is safe for coeliacs to eat unless it's been cooked with soy sauce, flour (although it could be rice flour) or breadcrumbs. If you ask for it salted it's likely to be safe.

In some parts of Japan you'll find crabs, depending on the season — king, hairy and snow crab. They are all delicious, but expensive in both restaurants and seafood markets. Cheap crab in the supermarket is probably just imitation made with wheat starch. You'll also find many different types of shrimp in Japan, all of which are good to cook and eat, or eaten raw as sushi. A packet of shrimp from the supermarket will add protein and colour to a dish of stir fried vegetables served with rice.

Meat

Not being great meat eaters, we didn't sample much pork, beef or lamb. In the main, these meats are quite expensive, especially compared to seafood and chicken. No doubt the quality is good, and they are generally only eaten in small amounts, such as thinly sliced for shabu shabu or in noodle dishes and on small barbecues. Steak with chips or mashed potato is readily available at many lunch venues and will be served plain and therefore gluten-free. Lamb seems to be most popular in Hokkaido. We avoided the horsemeat sushi, although it seemed quite popular in the south of Japan. You'll find at least six types of spam in Okinawa, and they are all gluten-free!

Tofu

Tofu is a great substitute for meat in stir fries, in salads and even for dessert. It is readily available in supermarkets, though we were lucky to be staying almost next door to a tofu factory in Itoman where we could buy it fresh and warm from 6 am. In Okinawa the factory (and supermarkets) sell several types of fresh tofu, whereas the tofu elsewhere is similar to the kind available in Australia.

Eggs

A large variety of eggs can be found in most supermarkets in Japan, and convenience stores often sell hard boiled eggs and packaged omelettes. How convenient! We cooked our own hard boiled eggs but they were so fresh they were often difficult to peel. Eggs make a handy meal as they can be hard boiled, fried, poached (we used the handy silicon cups from the hundred yen shop), scrambled or made into omelettes with vegetables incorporated or on the side.

Dairy

Hokkaido is well known for its dairy products. So you'll find delicious Hokkaido milk, butter, cream, cheese and yoghurt in shops all over Japan. Lots of different yoghurts are available, from plain low-fat to Greek yogurts. There are also several custardy desserts that are creamy, delicious and gluten-free — good eaten with fresh fruit or the jellied fruit (such as pears, nectarines, grapes) that are usually found on a nearby shelf.

Hokkaido icecream is to die for, very creamy and delicious. Icecream cones are easy to come by, but for gluten-free icecreams you'll need to ask for the ice cream to be scooped into a paper cup instead of a cone. Well known brands like Magnums, many of which are gluten-free, are easy to find. However our particular favourites were the MOW ice cream cups, found in many tourist venues and most supermarkets. They come in basic chocolate, green tea, berry and vanilla, with special flavours being released from time to time, and they are very cheap.

Photo Page 69: Crabs, Nijo Fish Market, Sapporo

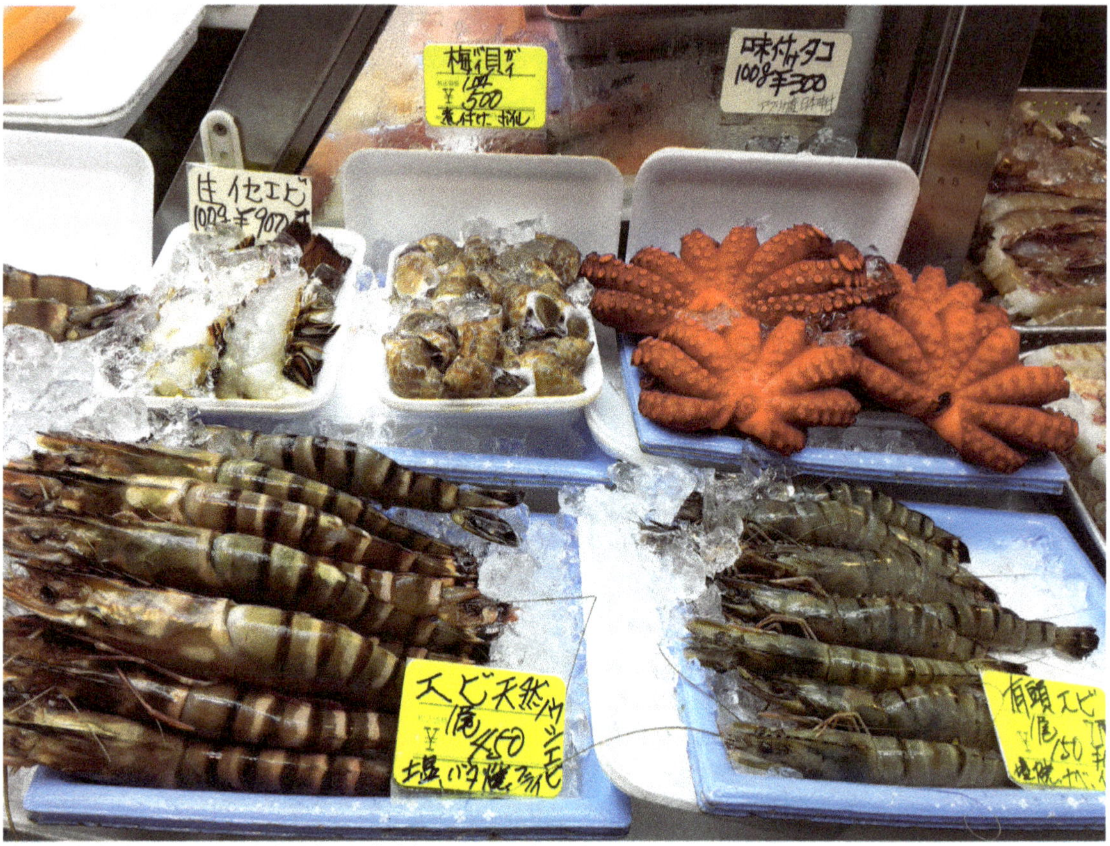

Above: Seafood in department store, Fukuoka; Below: Hard boiled eggs at supermarket, Aso Town

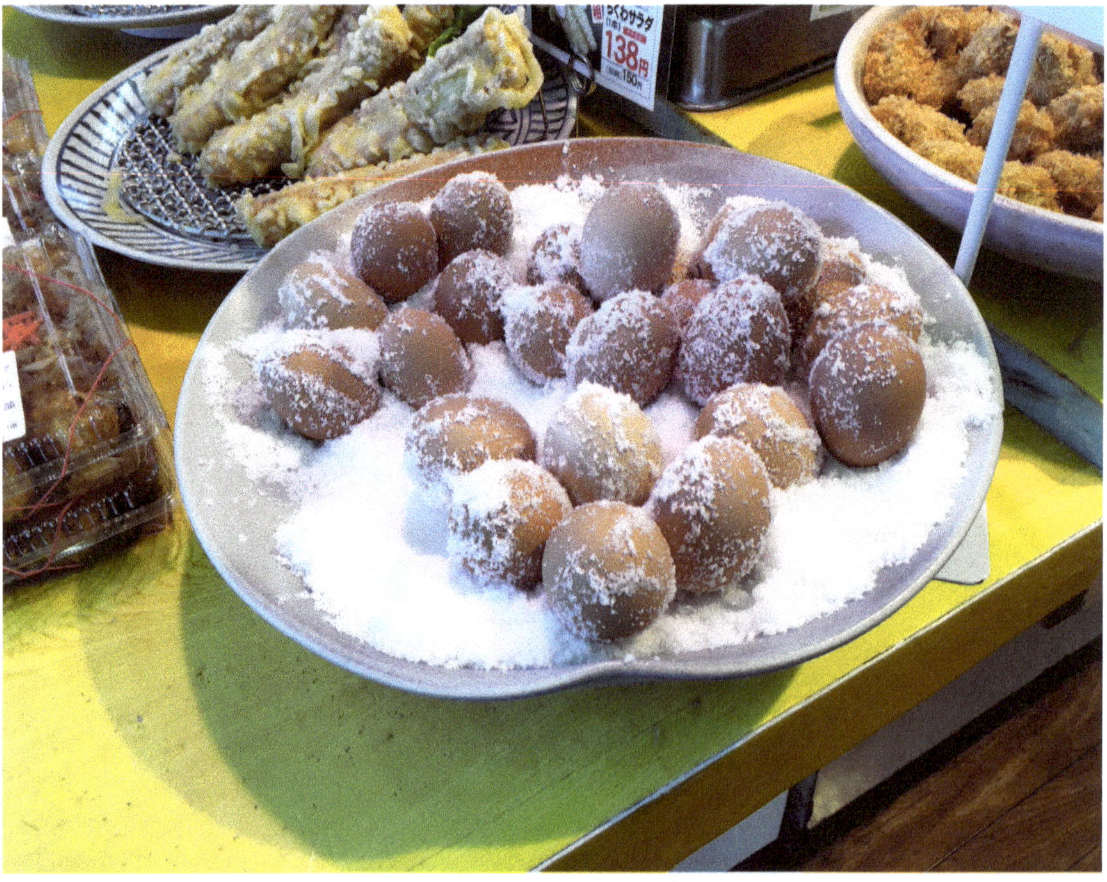

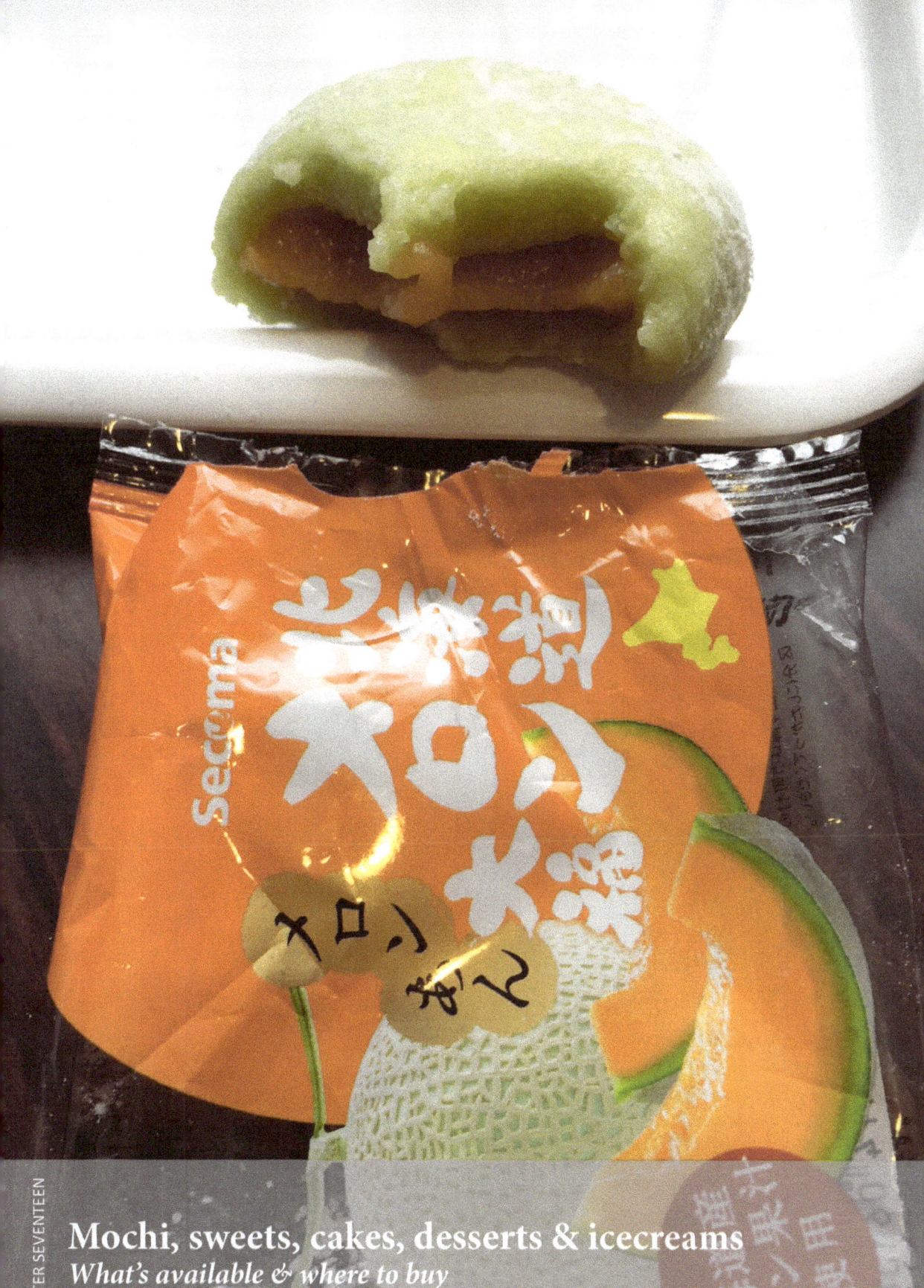

CHAPTER SEVENTEEN

Mochi, sweets, cakes, desserts & icecreams
What's available & where to buy

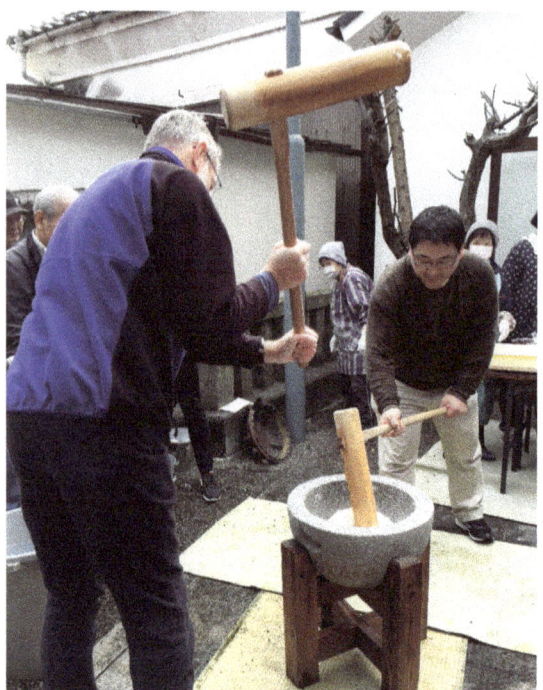

Above: Pounding rice for mochi, Beppu; Right: Stuffing mochi with red bean paste

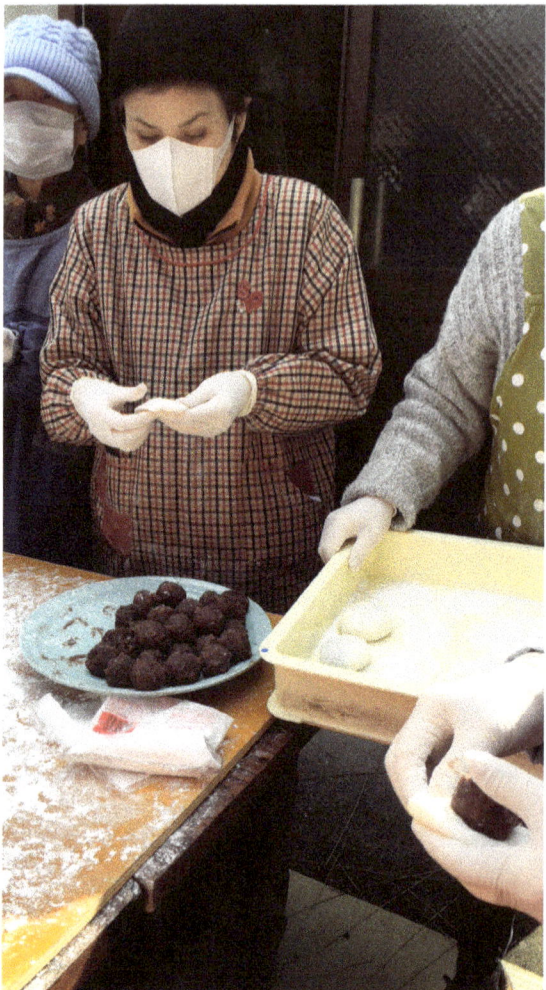

Left: Gluten-free kutchen, Roppongi Hills; Below: Zenzai red bean & shaved ice

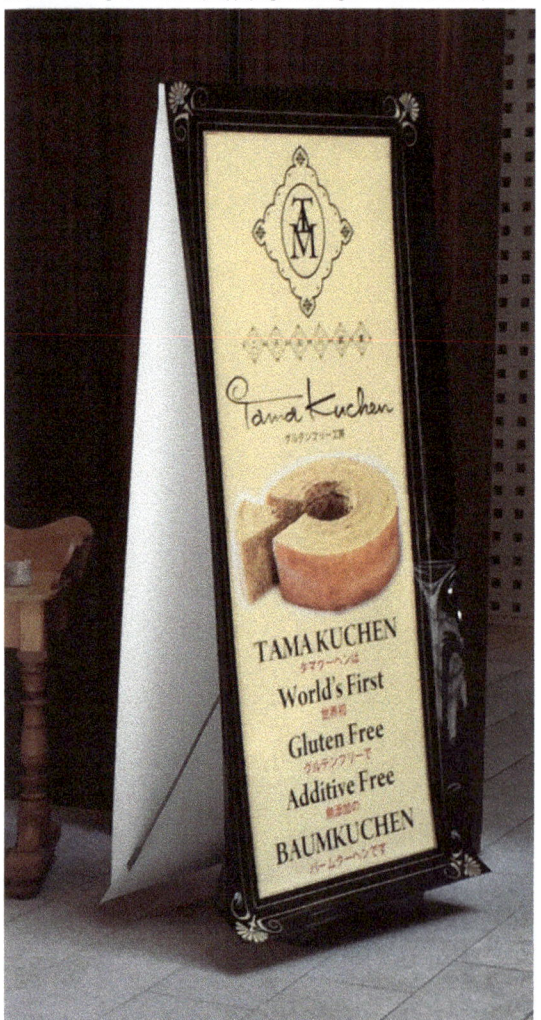

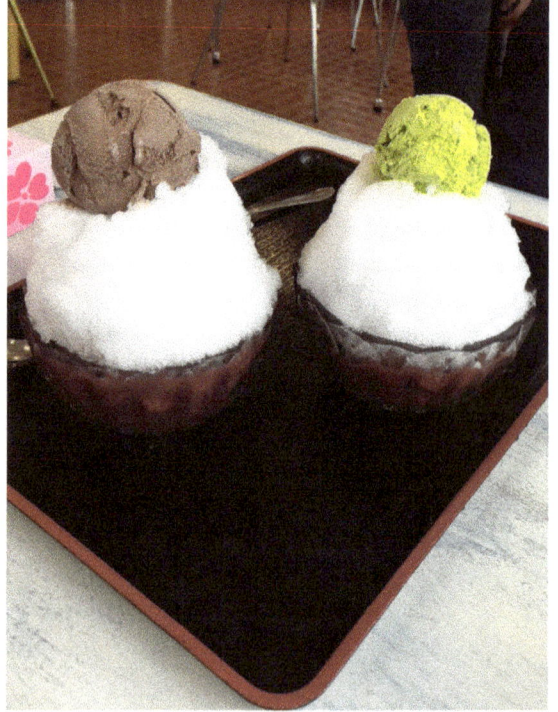

MOCHI, SWEETS, CAKES, DESSERTS & ICECREAMS: What's available & where to buy

Mochi

Mochi — pounded rice balls with sweet fillings — are sometimes, but not always, gluten-free. Our local Japanese cake shop, Ishimura, in Fukuoka, stocked a beautiful array of mochi and cakes. The staff searched for products that didn't contain wheat and found some mochi (including chestnut ones) and a variety of marshmellows that were suitable. One day, in Beppu, we were really fortunate to come across a community mochi-making event, and were even invited try our hand at pounding the rice and stuffing the mochi with red bean paste.

If you read the labels carefully you'll be rewarded with some beautiful mochi — including red bean paste, custard, horse chestnut, chocolate mint, mango, musk melon and gingko. Our favourites had whole fruits like a strawberry or a small sweet mandarin (mikan) inside. While most mochi are made with pounded white rice, green mochi with rice coloured with matcha (green tea), are also common. Mochi make good snacks when you're on the go — including the frozen white or pink icecream mochi from convenience stores or supermarkets.

Sweets & cakes

At festivals you'll find an abundance of bananas on sticks, coated with chocolate or other sweet things. And be sure to check out the 'omiyage' (souvenirs), as some of the sweet ones are gluten-free. Dried persimmons are to die for! However, 'wagashi', the beautifully coloured small traditional Japanese sweets served at tea ceremonies, are best avoided. They don't have ingredients listed but most times we were told they contained ingredients that weren't gluten-free.

Most cakes made in Japan are, of course, not gluten-free and most bakeries are French style. It's hardly worth the effort of going into the bakery section of a supermarket or into a cake shop, unless you want to investigate their mochi. We did find a few places that sold gluten-free cakes. There are at least two in Tokyo. One was Otaco in Asakusa, which specialises in various flavours of gluten-free cakes such as earl grey, walnut and raisin, green tea and mocha, made with rice flour. The other was a small shop in the Roppongi Hills area that sold a gluten-free version of 'kutchen', the German layer cake, correctly called 'baumkuchen', meaning 'tree cake' after the characteristic rings seen when sliced. Wheat flour kutchen are popular in Japan and can be found in most bakeries. As you'd expect, products in both shops were very expensive! A small gluten-free restaurant in Niseko also sold takeaway frozen chiffon cakes and cookies.

Desserts

Some of the chocolate-based Godiva desserts at Lawson Station convenience stores are gluten-free, and you're sure to find something for dessert in any convenience store or supermarket if you look at the creme caramels, rice puddings, creamy desserts, yoghurts and tofu. They can be paired with icecream and/or fresh or jellied fruit to make some lovely desserts. Alternatively grab some chocolates, mochi or an icecream. Red bean desserts called 'zenzai' have a soup base made from adzuki (red beans), sugar/fruits and small mochi. The Okinawan version either has shaved ice on top of the soup or is simply made from coloured shaved ice and icecream.

Icecreams

Most convenience stores and supermarkets stock a range of stick icecreams such as Magnum and Lady Borden brands, as well as icecream mochi and a good variety of bucket icecreams such as the ubiquitous NorgenVass. We even bought special buckwheat (soba) icecreams at the Soba Museum near Nagano and sake flavoured icecreams at Saijo near Hiroshima. The best value and nicest icecreams are the MOW brand of bucket icecreams (see Chapter 16), which are handy to keep a stock of in the freezer if you're staying in an Airbnb. But if you buy them while out and about, don't forget to ask for a spoon!

Icecreams are readily available at all tourist places in Japan. Just indicate you want a cup instead of a cone. It's worth trying out some very unusual flavours. At the Happiness Dairy near Ikeda in Hokkaido we tried sesame, pumpkin, potato and rhubarb-haskap!

Photo Page 73: Rock melon mochi, Hokkaido

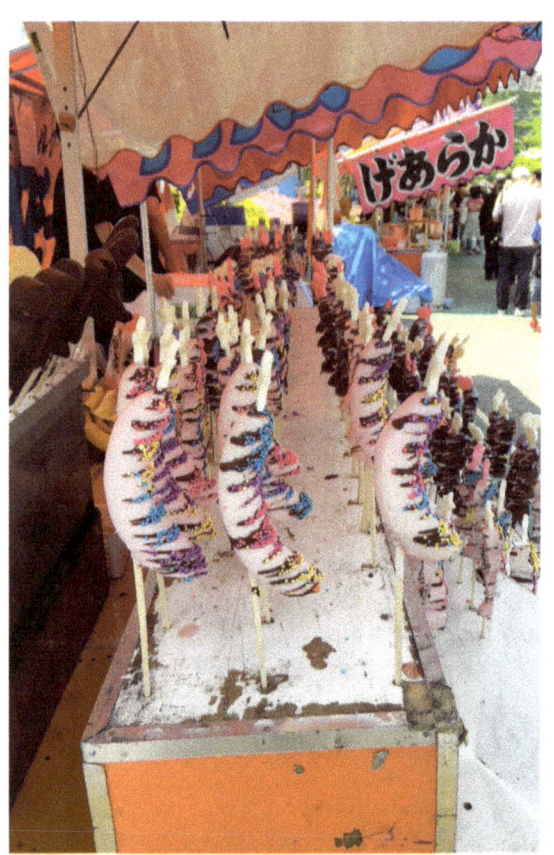
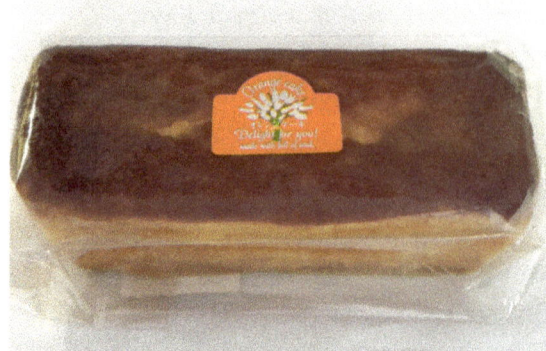

Above: Gluten-free cake from Otaco, Asakusa, Tokyo

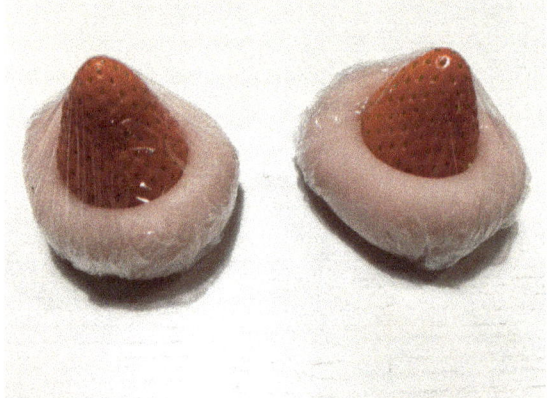

Above: Bananas at festival in Tokyo; Below: Lime omiyage (souvenirs), Kyushu

Above: Strawberry mochi, Takumatsu

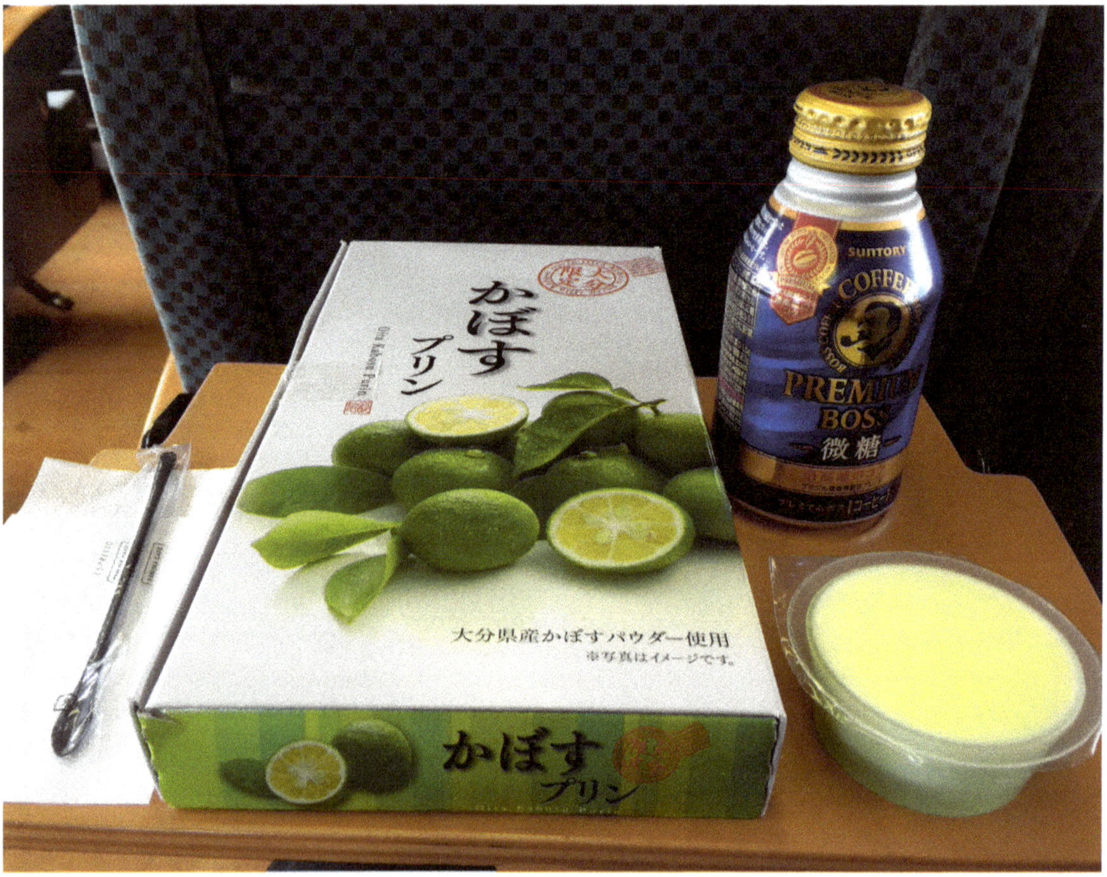

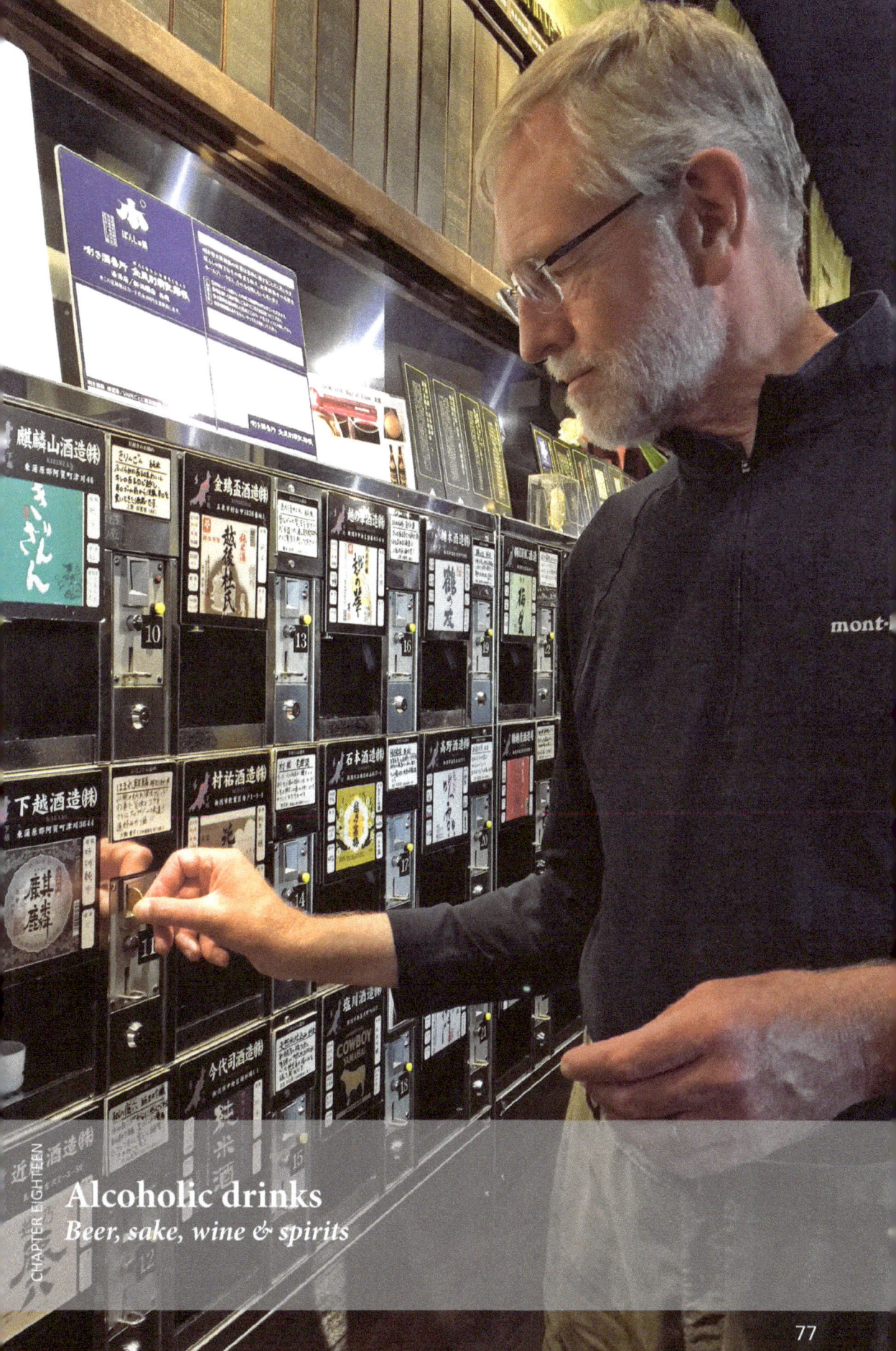

Alcoholic drinks
Beer, sake, wine & spirits

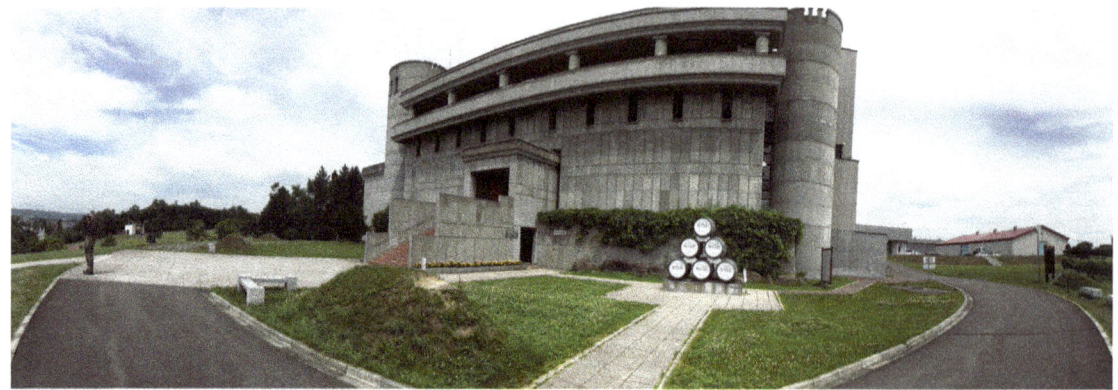

Above: Ikeda Wine Castle, Hokkaido; Below: Sake and sparkling sake in 300 ml bottles from convenience store

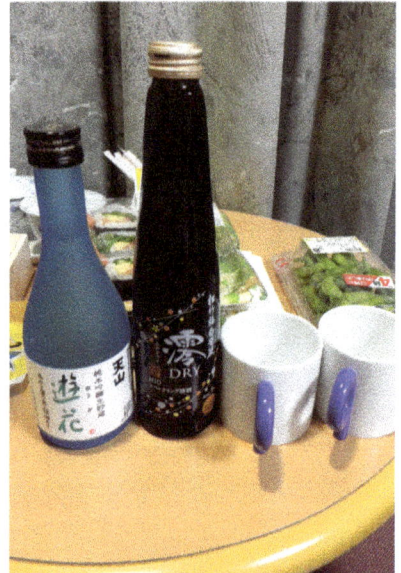
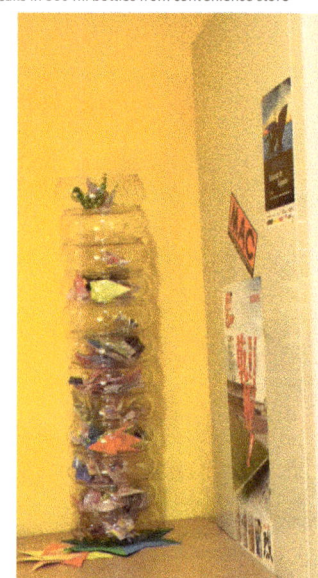
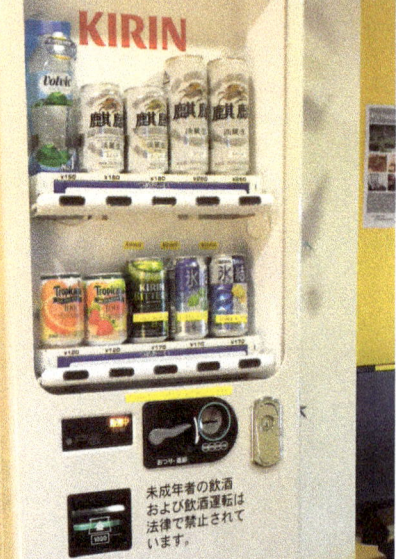

Below: Sake sampling, Imaya Tsukasa Sake Brewery, Niigata   Above: Drink vending machine in hotel

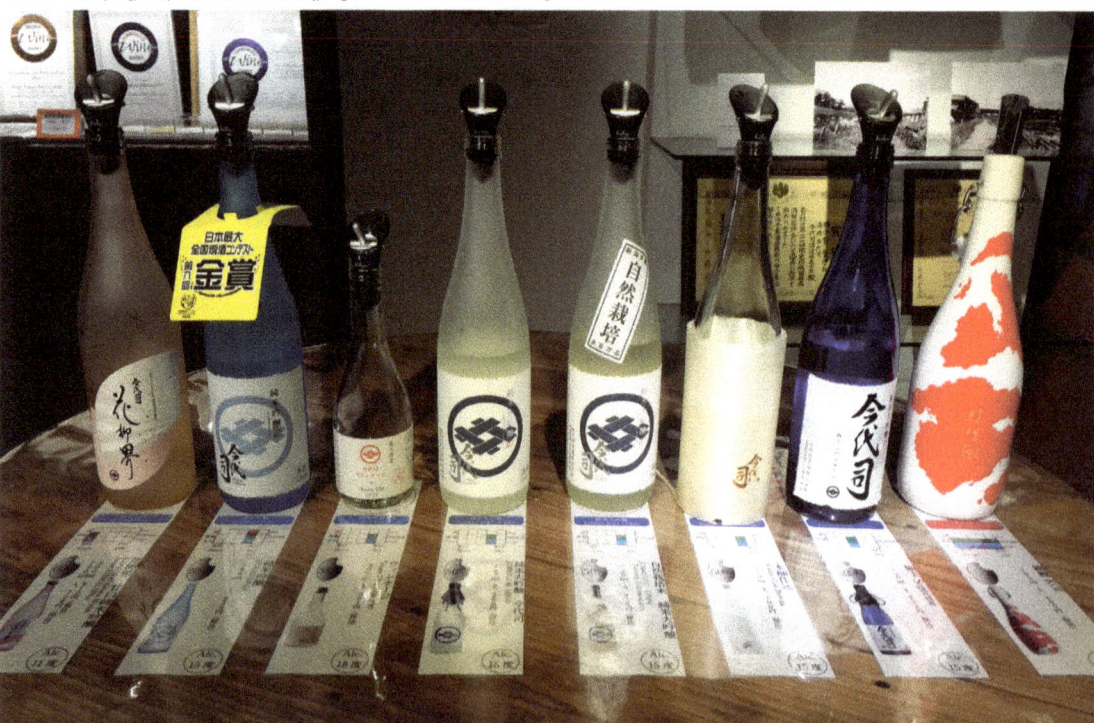

ALCOHOLIC DRINKS: Beer, sake, wine & spirits

Beer

Beer is very popular throughout Japan and the country produces many excellent beers — though, alas, we didn't find any gluten-free varieties. It is similar in price to beer in Australia and is sold in cans of various sizes up to 3 litres! Even if your friends are drinking beer, there are plenty of alternatives available at restaurants, pubs, hotels and at events — although it would probably be best to avoid going to one of the many beer festivals! That said, a tour of the Asahi Factory in Fukuoka was a great experience, despite not being able to drink the samples at the end of the tour (soft drinks were also provided).

Sake

Sake, or Japanese rice wine made from rice, water and koji mold, is an excellent alternative to beer. It's readily available in warm, cold and sparkling varieties and in many different sizes of both bottles and cartons. We carried our own lightweight ceramic sake cups with us. So it meant we were always prepared!

Like wine, sake comes in different types (from dry to sweet), different qualities and there are regional differences, seemingly due to differences in water quality. Eighty per cent of Japanese sake is 'table sake', made with rice polished to a minimum of 70% (i.e. at least 30% has been milled away). The remaining twenty per cent is premium. The top quality sakes (jumai-daiginjo-shu) have at least 50% milled away. Along with the alcohol content, this number appears on every sake that you buy — simply remember that the lower the percentage, the better the quality.

Because sake is the traditional drink of Japan, there are lots of sake breweries to visit for a tour. They can be recognised by the 'sugidama' (cedar twig balls) hanging above the front door. Traditionally, these were green and hung to announce that fresh sake had been made; when they turned brown, the sake was ready to drink. If you come across 'new sake', have a taste. It's milky with sediment and has quite a different flavour. Saijo, known as Sake Town, located near Hiroshima, boasts eight breweries in the one area and is definitely worth a visit.

Photo Page 79: Sampling sake at the Sake Museum at Niigata Station

One of the highlights of Niigata is the Sake Museum, where you can not only learn a lot about sake, but you can also sample over 100 types of sake. For 500 yen, you can taste five different ones. It's a good way to find out which type suits you best (dry or sweet) and perhaps choose which to buy for dinner.

Wine

Wine is available in convenience stores and supermarkets in Japan, along with liquor stores and the Kaldi Coffee Farm outlets. The choice is good, with plenty of Australian, Chilean, Argentinian and other imported wines available, as well as some Japanese ones. Compared to Australia, the prices are quite a bit cheaper because of lower taxes. The Ikeda Wine Castle in Hokkaido is worth visiting, as it showcases local vintages and doubles as a wine research centre where they are investigating grape varieties suitable for winter snow.

Spirits

Spirits are also cheaper in Japan than in Australia, because of the taxes. There's a wide range of mixed drinks that are gluten-free and available in supermarkets and vending machines — such as gin and tonic and vodka and whiskey highballs. Both whiskey and beer were available on tap at the baseball game we attended in Yokohama.

Shochu is another great alternative for coeliacs. It usually has an alcohol content around 25%, so is stronger than wine and sake but not as strong as whiskey or vodka. It is made using rice, barley, sweet potatoes or buckwheat, but all are distilled and therefore gluten-free. Shochu is usually drunk 'on the rocks.'

Awamori is a much stronger brew (30-40%) and is unique to Okinawa and usually drunk with water and ice. Awamori is made from long-grain Thai rice and the price varies with age. The liquor is usually aged in traditional clay pots containing a habu snake, whose poison becomes safe with time due to the alcohol. Tofuyo — fermented tofu aged in awamori — has a taste like blue cheese and is a delicious accompaniment for alcoholic drinks.

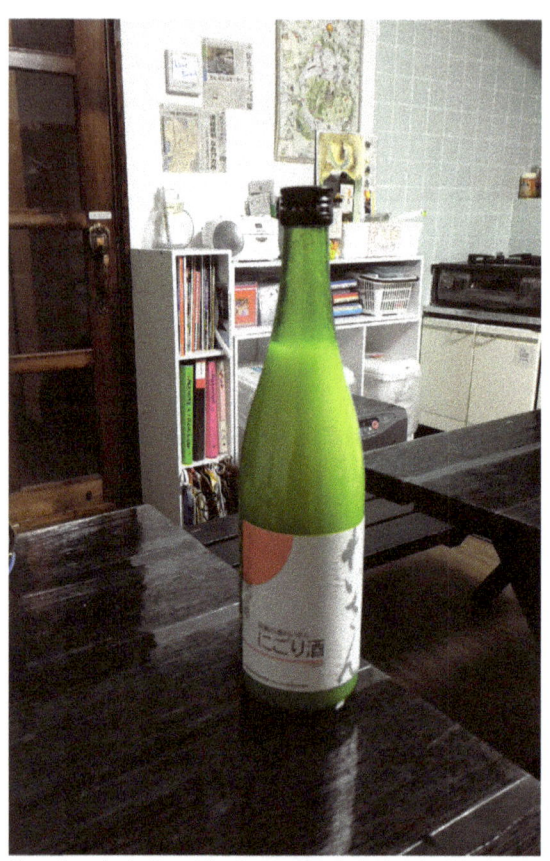
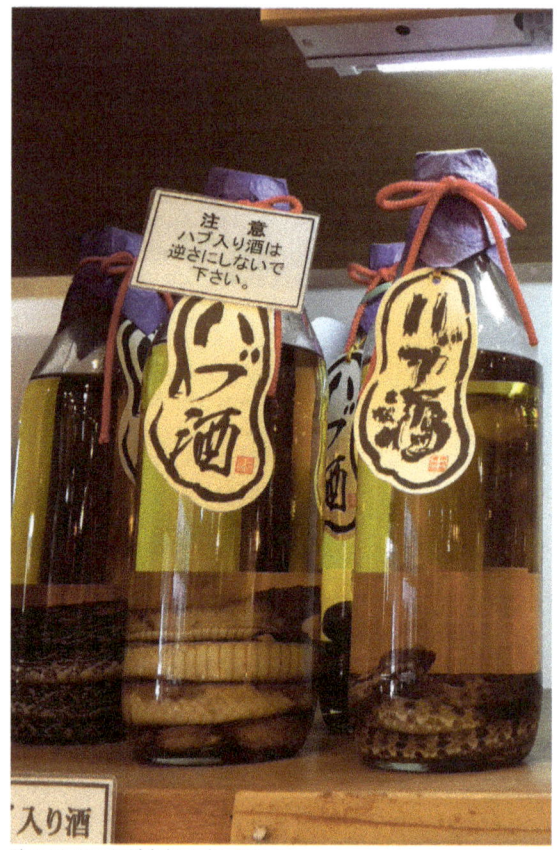

Above: New sake, Aso Town; Below: Customers' shochu bottles in bar, Fukuoka

Above: Awamori with habu snakes, Okinawa

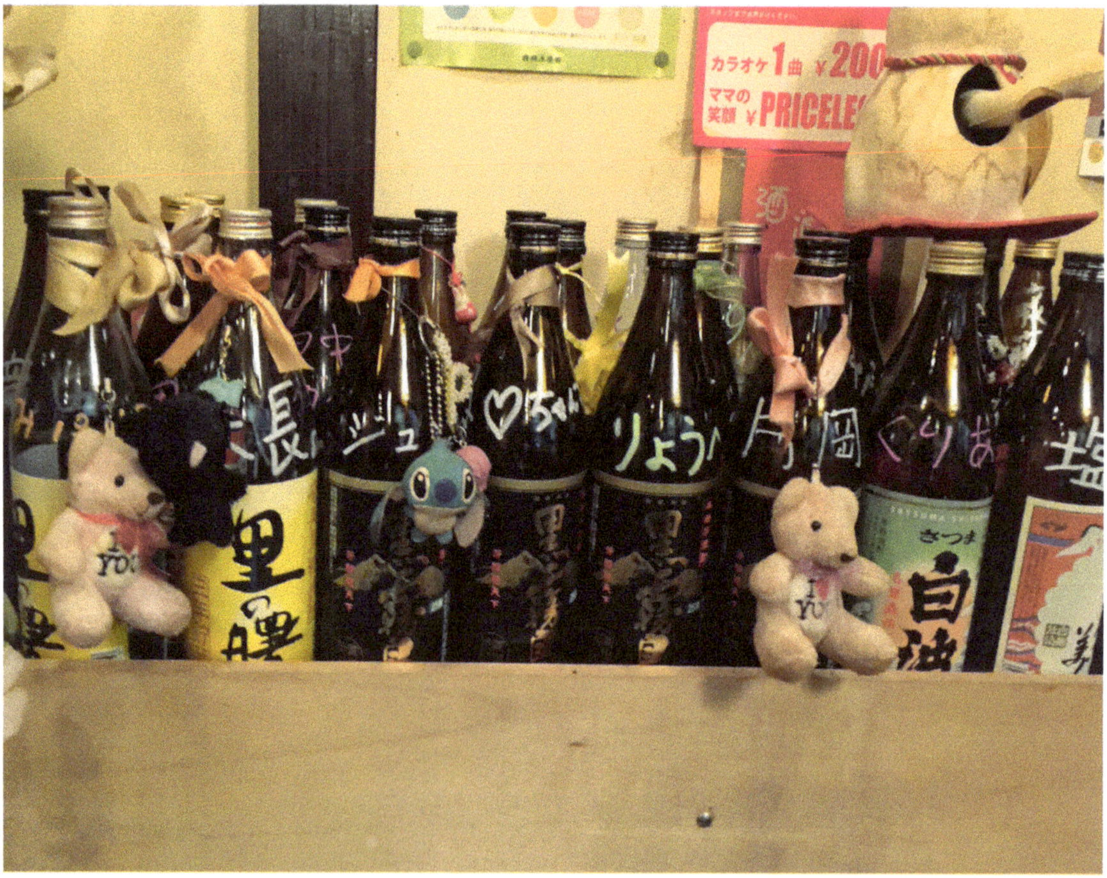

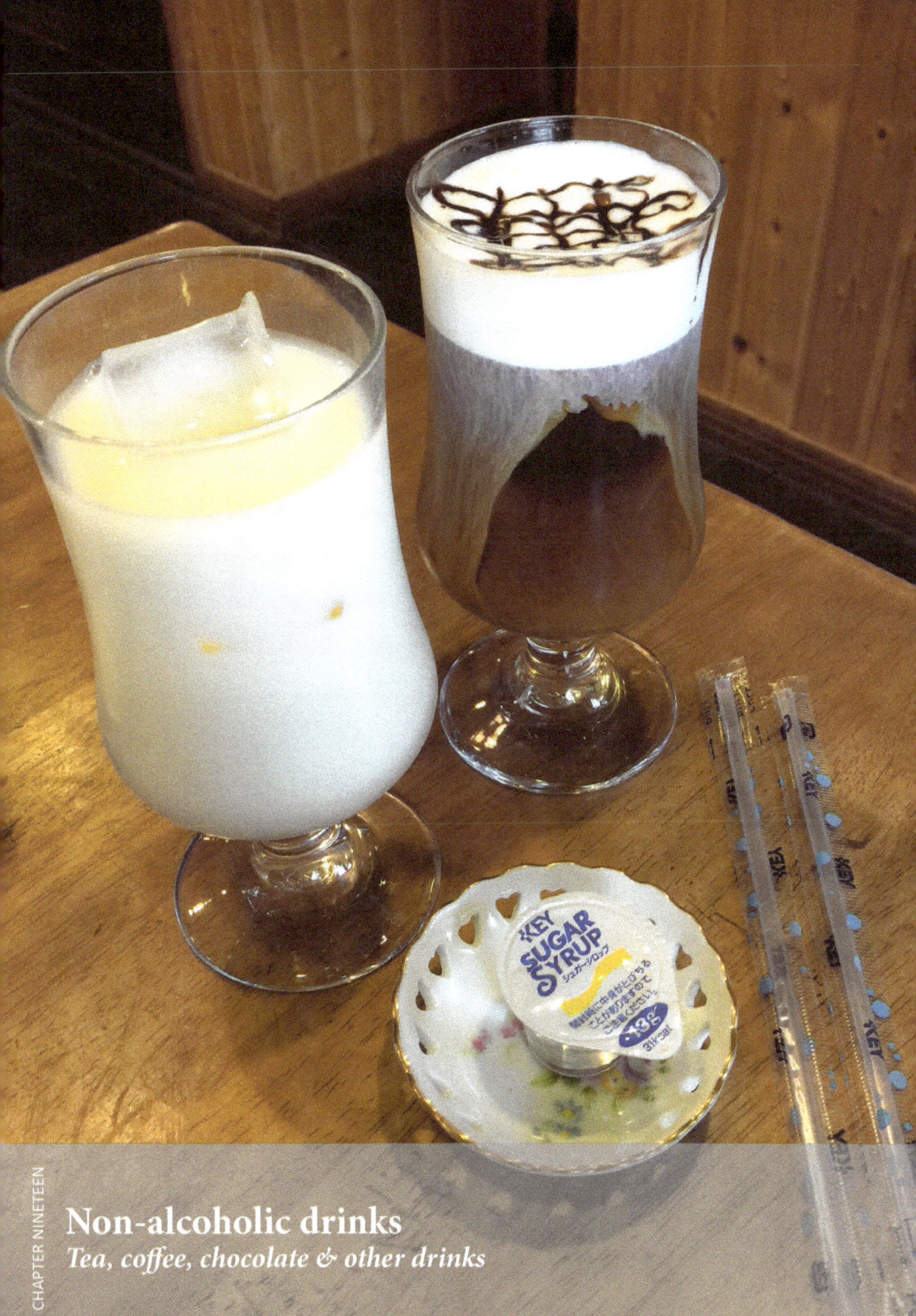

Non-alcoholic drinks
Tea, coffee, chocolate & other drinks

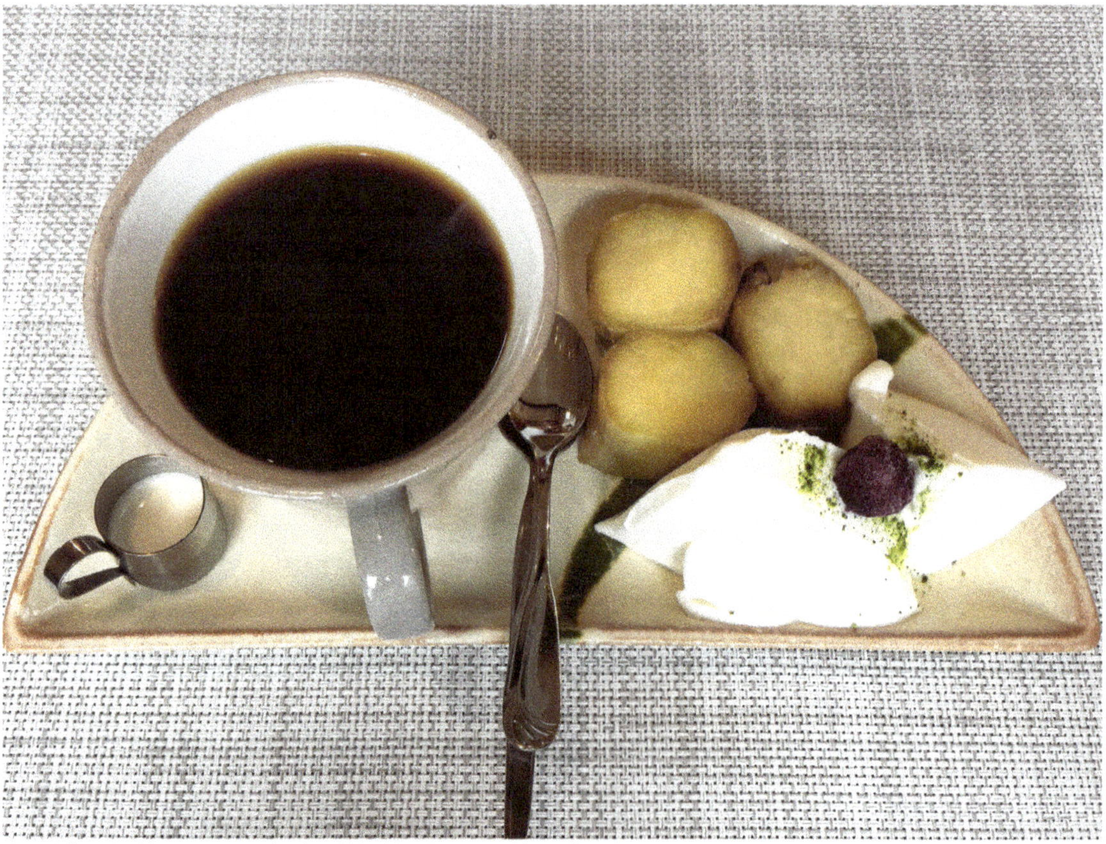

Above: Coffee with cold sweet potatoes and yoghurt, Nikko; Below: Green tea and dessert, Tsuruoka

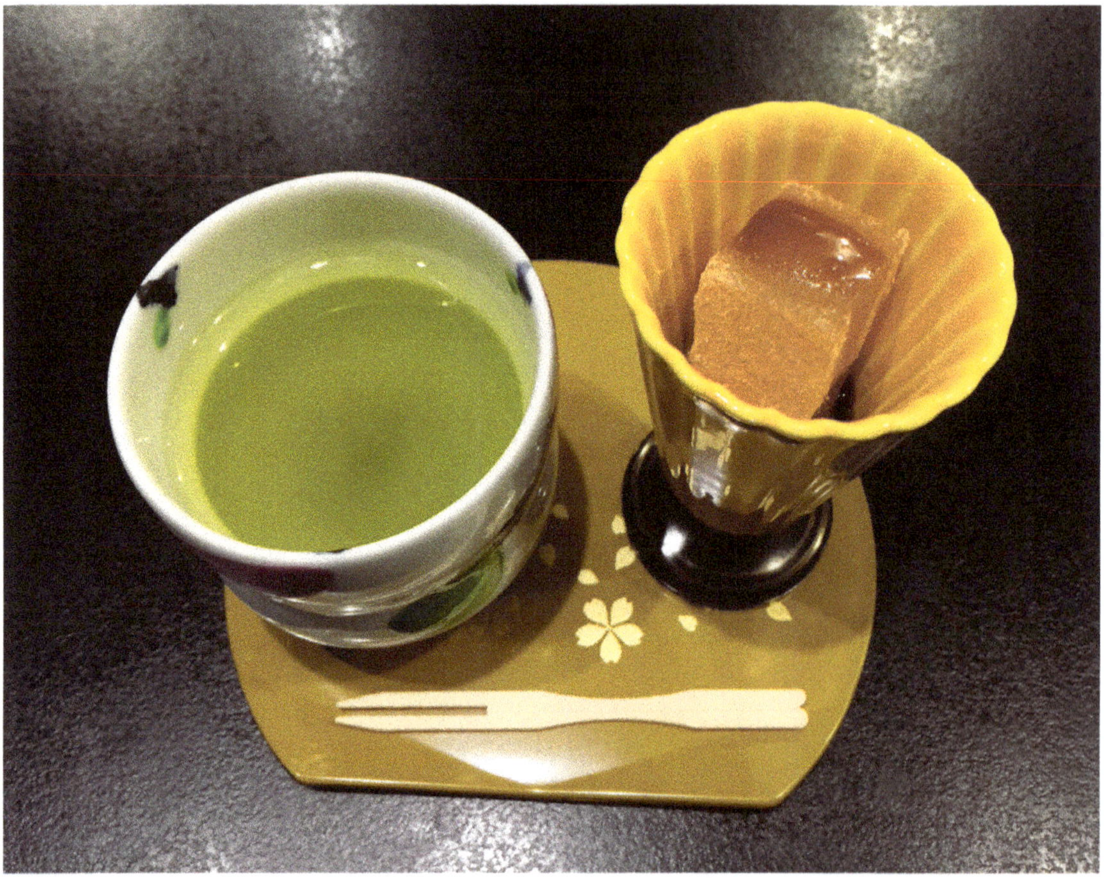

NON-ALCOHOLIC DRINKS: Tea, coffee, chocolate & other drinks

Tea

Japan is well known for its tea ceremonies. These are incredibly complicated rituals, steeped in tradition and ceremony. If you get a chance to take part in one, it's well worth it. We took a class is Tokyo, organised by our Airbnb host just at the time that Airbnb 'Experiences' were newly launched. We had an interpreter who also took photos so that we could concentrate on the class. Often when you buy tea at a temple, you'll be served with green tea in a similarly formal manner, along with traditional Japanese sweets called 'wagashi' — which probably won't be gluten-free.

For making tea at home, plenty of green and black teas are available to buy as packets of leaf tea, tea bags and matcha (powdered green tea), in convenience stores and supermarkets. Both have huge sections of hot and cold ready-to-drink teas in either plastic or metal cup-sized containers. You'll also find larger bottles of flavoured tea (e.g. lemon, mango, green) in the fridge section alongside the bottles of water and soft drinks.

Coffee

Hot and cold coffees are kept in separate compartments in convenience stores, along with hot/cold teas and chocolate drinks. Be warned — most Japanese drinks are a lot sweeter than we are used to in Australia, unless marked as 'no sugar', 'unsweetened' or 'low sugar'.

Coffee shops abound in Japan. There are plenty of Starbucks around major railway stations and in the cities and they serve the same range of over-sweet concoctions (our opinion!) as weekly or seasonal specials made with a multitude of ingredients including syrups. Still, it may be your thing and they are bound to have some varieties that are gluten-free.

You can buy reasonable quality coffees from convenience stores (to take away or drink in), usually made from a machine at the counter, but the best coffee has to be found by trial and error at coffee shops. We found a place in the main street of Nikko that featured potato dishes and they served a nice black coffee with cold, cooked sweet potatoes and yoghurt. It might sound strange, but it was so good — and gluten-free — that we returned for more on another day!

Many Airbnbs have devices for making filtered coffee at home. However, we found the most convenient were the drip coffee bags. You can buy these in packets of five, ten or more. They come in individual sealed packets (like some tea bags) and use a variety of cleverly folded filtering devices that sit on top of a cup so that you can pour boiling water through the coffee. The more expensive brands are the best quality and we even found drip bags of the Italian Lavazza brand in suburban Fukuoka.

Chocolate

Chocolate milk, as well as other flavours, abounds in larger supermarkets, in cartons of up to two litres. Both hot and cold chocolate drinks are found in convenience stores, supermarkets and in vending machines. We highly recommend the Godiva brand of hot chocolates (and superior coffees) bought over the counter at Lawson Station stores. You might find that these, like all chocolate drinks in Japan, are overly sweet. Occasionally, you'll also find hot chocolate drinks made by adding particulate chocolate to hot milk.

Other drinks

Look out for the yoghurt drinks in convenience stores and supermarkets as they are usually delicious. The Seven Eleven plain yoghurt drink is great and they have a range of flavours that often feature small chunks of various fruits. Of course, there are lots and lots of soft drinks and fruit juices to choose from and they are all likely to be gluten-free like the yoghurt drinks. Note, however, that mixer drinks, such as tonic water, may be hard to find, or located in the alcohol section of a supermarket, should you fancy a gin and tonic now and then.

Some of the nicest fruit drinks we encountered were at a palm conservation area on the island of Ishigaki in the Yaeyama Islands. The vendor had a fire going to extract sugar juice from raw sugar cane, which he blended with fresh guava and/or pineapple.

Photo Page 81: Cold milk and hot chocolate, Tateyama

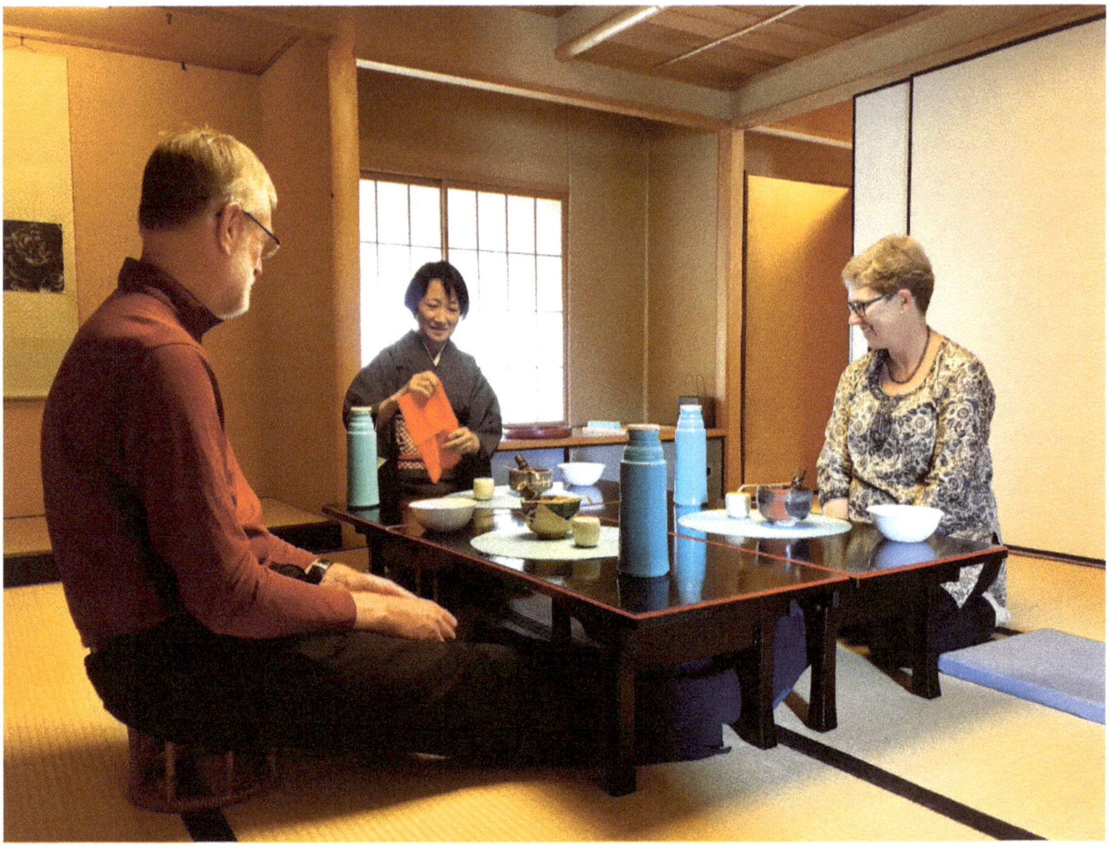

Above: Tea ceremony, Tokyo; Below: Vending machine with hot (red) and cold (blue) drinks

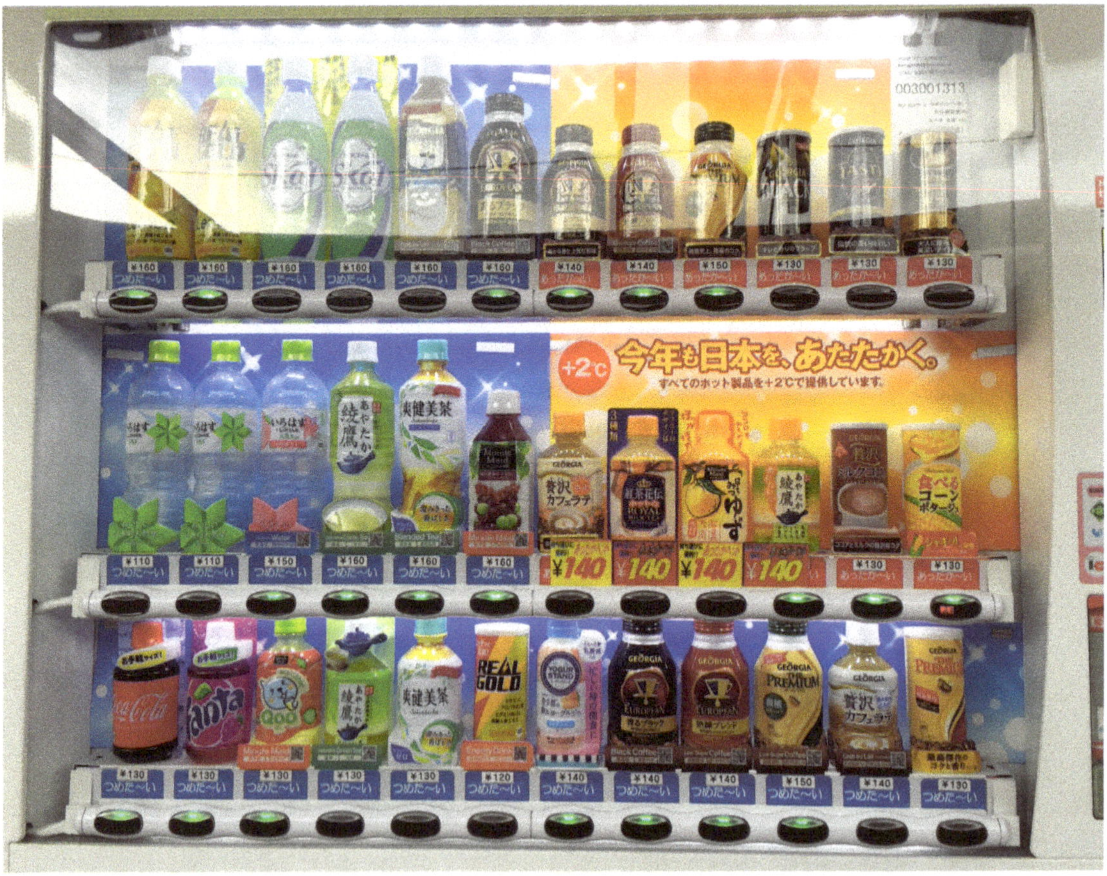

84

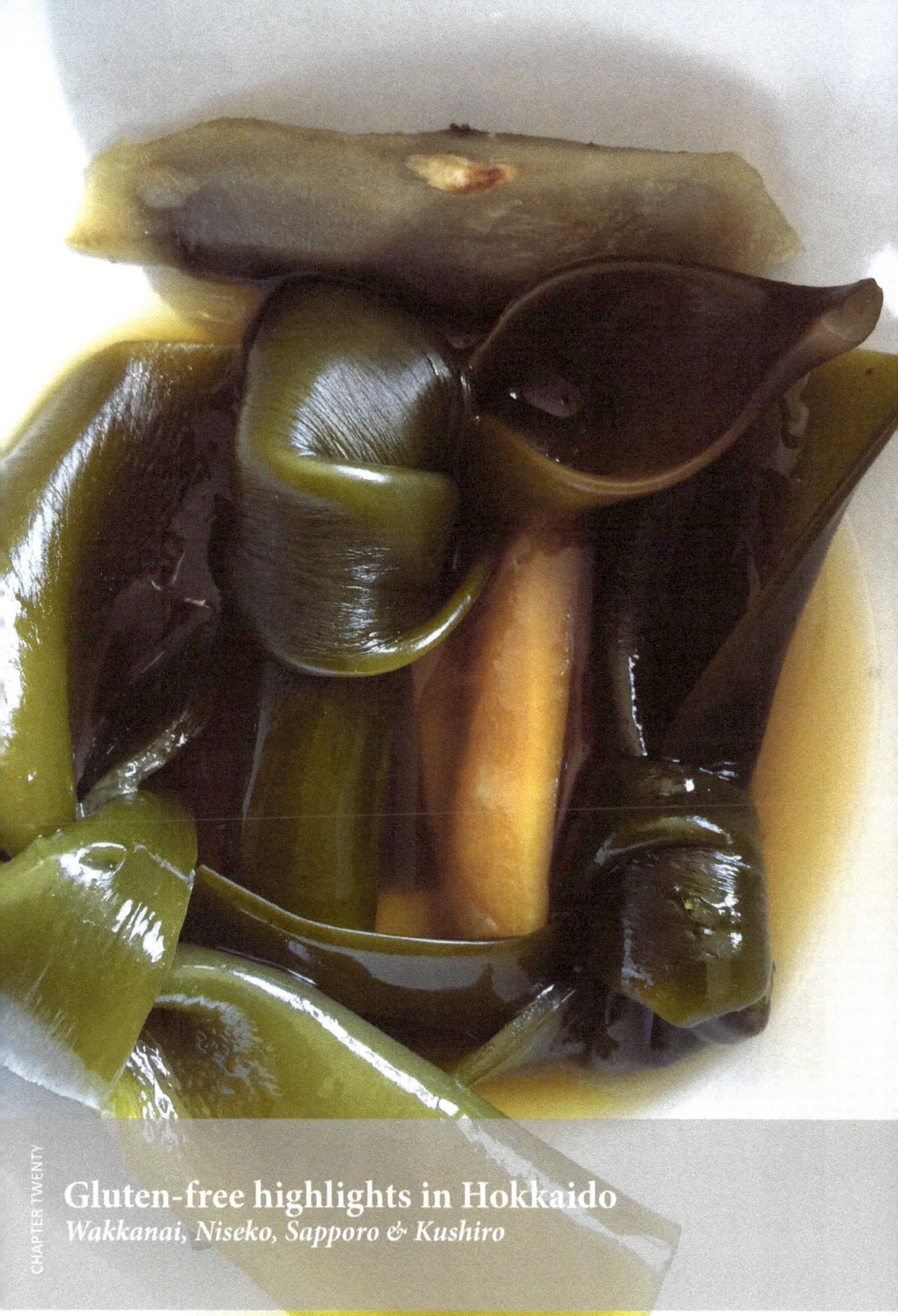

Gluten-free highlights in Hokkaido
Wakkanai, Niseko, Sapporo & Kushiro

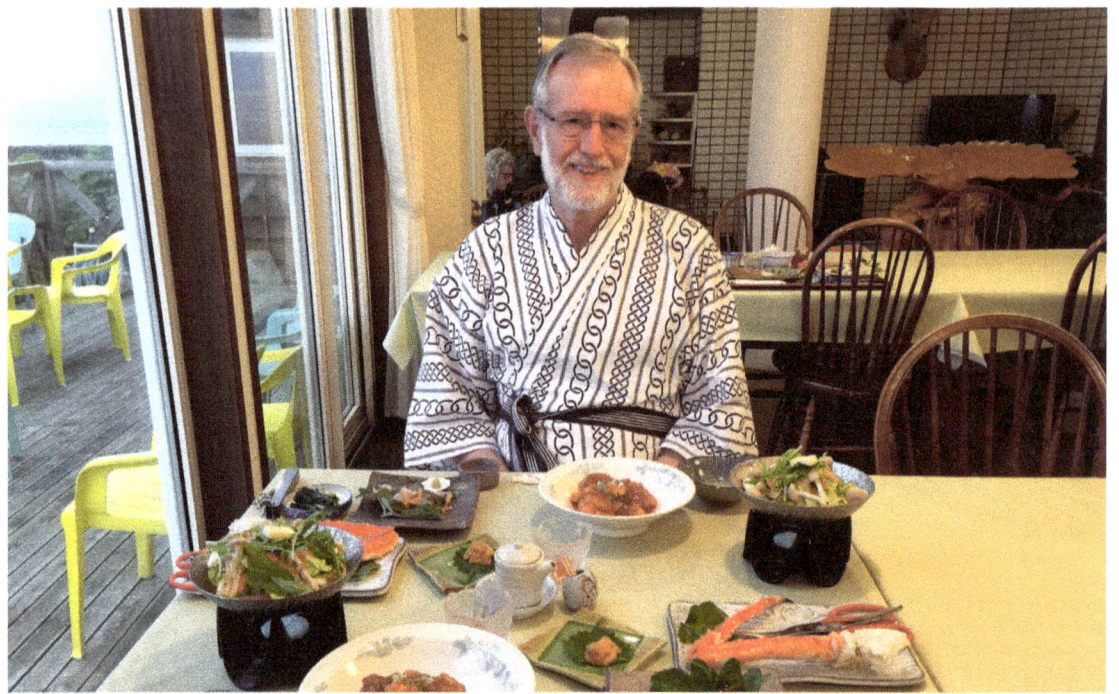
Above: Meal at Pension Arumeria, Wakkanai; Below: Pension Arumeria, Wakkanai

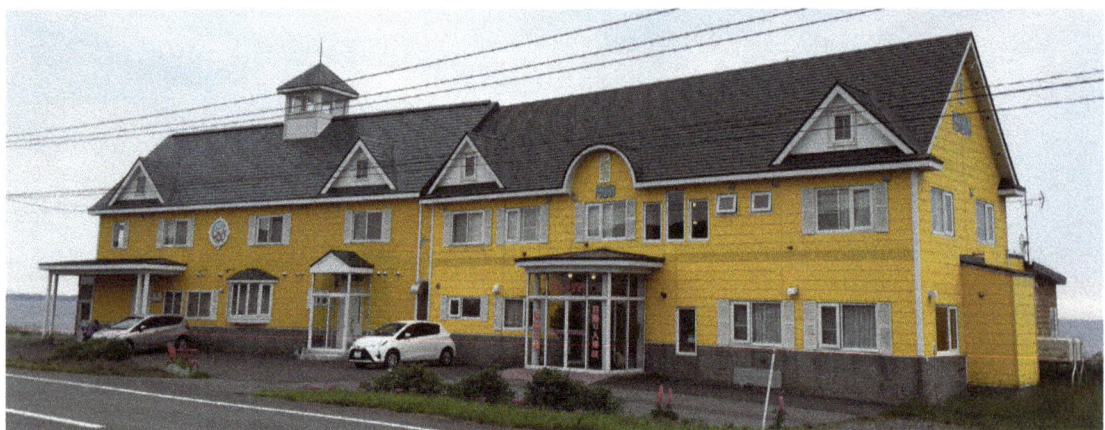

Below Left: Gluten-free Cafe Yukiya, Niseko; Below Right: Desserts at Cafe Yukiya

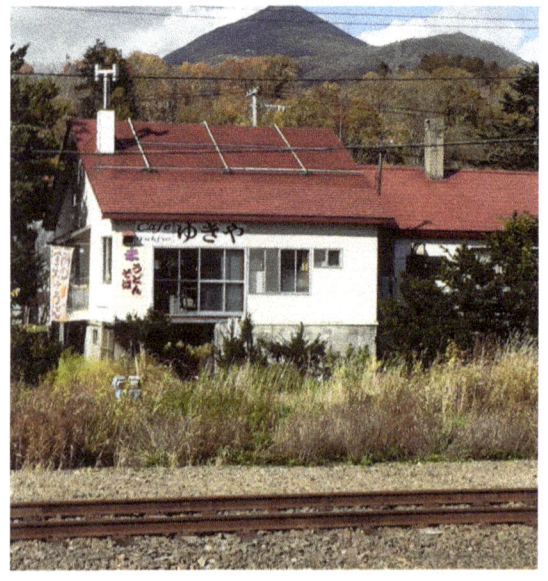
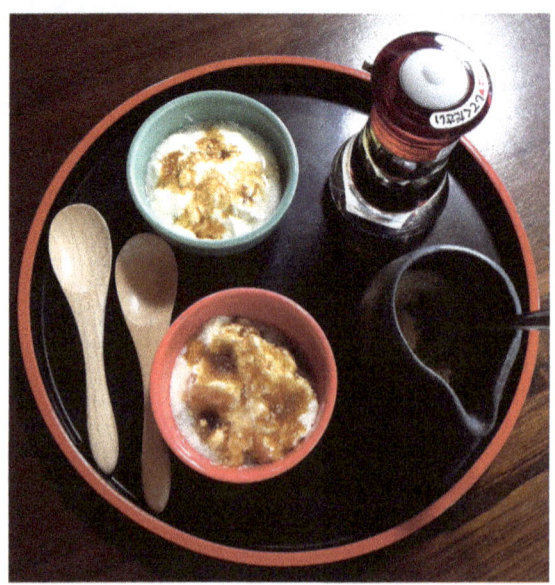

GLUTEN-FREE HIGHLIGHTS IN HOKKAIDO: Wakkanai, Niseko, Sapporo & Kushiro

Wakkanai

The food at the gorgeous yellow Pension Arumeria, set right on the beach in the middle of nowhere about fifteen kilometres out of Wakkanai, was utterly amazing. We stayed for the best part of a week and we chose to have all breakfasts and most dinners included. When we checked in, we explained about the gluten-free requirement and the staff went out of their way to prepare all our meals accordingly.

If you like seafood, then this gem in Wakkanai will be all you hope for and more. Every day the food became more and more interesting and (mostly!) delicious. Having already travelled the length and breadth of Japan by then, this is quite some statement. The meals (or rather the components, since they were huge multi-dish affairs) included pickled sea cucumber, octopus shabu-shabu, octopus head, octopus gills, three types of clams, three types of prawns, whelks, squid, sea urchin roe, salmon roe, king crab, hairy crab, two types of scallops, and some very unusual fish such as flying fish and karei (right-eyed flounder) which has a jelly-like consistency. There were also curries and vegetables such as okra, daikon (white radish), mushrooms and seaweeds.

Niseko

Halfway up the hill from Niseko station to our cottage (a three kilometre hike), we found a lovely restaurant called Suttu's Restaurant Kagra. It was a very pleasant place with a good range of gluten-free meals on offer. We had seafood on rice and fish but vowed to return and try some of the other dishes. This wasn't meant to be, however, because we found an actual dedicated gluten-free restaurant just on the other (mountain) side of the railway station and it happened to be open on our only other available free day. Called Cafe Yukiya, the place is tiny and intimate, and all meals are gluten- and casein-free. The menu was interesting and included several hot-pots with chicken, duck or ham, a germinated brown rice porridge (called 'medicine caterpillar') and some beautiful desserts made from soy yoghurt with rough dark sugar sprinkled on top.

Sapporo

You'll find many good restaurants in Sapporo, but if you want a classy place with a comprehensive buffet menu that includes a wealth of gluten-free options, then Tsuruga, upstairs and opposite the Former Government Building, is the place to go. You need to book ahead via their website (in English) for one of the two lunchtime sittings. Another absolute highlight was the discovery of a Tonden restaurant close to where we stayed in one of the suburbs of Sapporo. We had various groups of friends staying with us and it was not only cheap but catered to everyone's various dietary requirements.

Kushiro

We were fortunate to come across various kelp-harvesting activities in Hokkaido, firstly on the Rausu coast near Shiretoko, where kelp was being pulled from boats and hauled onto trestle tables for washing. We saw the huge fronds being laid out on the gravelly beaches and learnt that the cold misty conditions were ideal for the gradual process of turning the kelp into a semi-dry state. The conditions were certainly ideal — we had fog every day during the whole month we drove around Hokkaido! We also saw fronds hanging in sheds, being dried with big fans, their doors open wide and their owners waiting patiently.

Back in Rausu there was an interesting photographic exhibition about the history of kelp harvesting in the area. Kelp, like all seaweeds, is gluten-free, and is incorporated into many Japanese dishes. Konbu, the finished kelp product, is used especially for flavouring stocks. However, it can also be eaten as a vegetable when relatively fresh. We later came across more harvesting and packaging activities along the Kiritappu coast ('kiri' meaning foggy), where one of the kelp farmers kindly gave us a small bunch of konbu to take home. We presented it to our host at the Yasumizaka Guest House in Kushiro and were pleasantly surprised when she dished up a konbu and vegetable dish for breakfast the following day. What a highlight — to see kelp processing from start to finish!

Photo Page 85: Konbu cooked by our guest house host, Kushiro

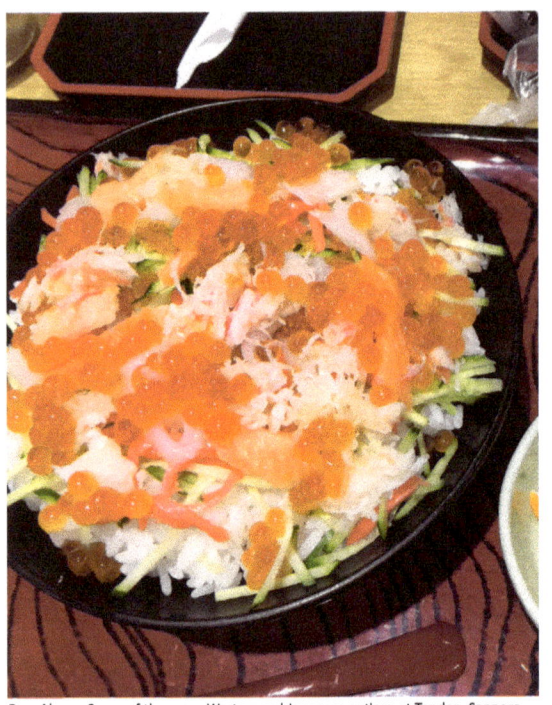
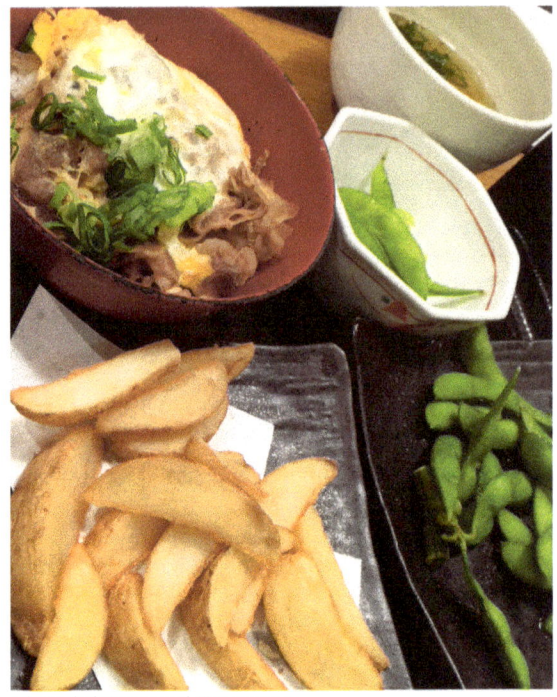

Row Above: Some of the many Western and Japanese options at Tonden, Sapporo

Below: Kelp drying on gravel, Kiritappu coast

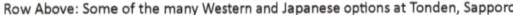

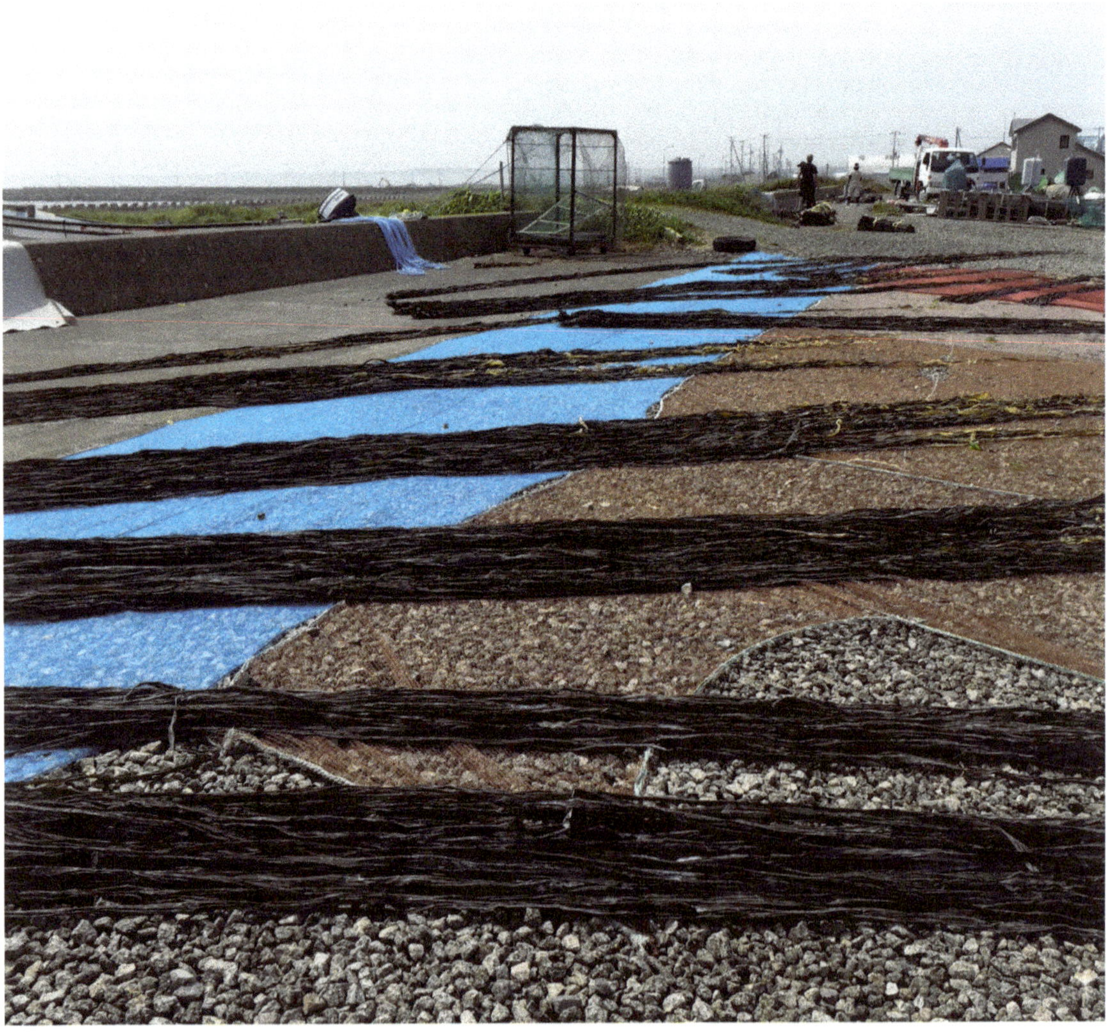

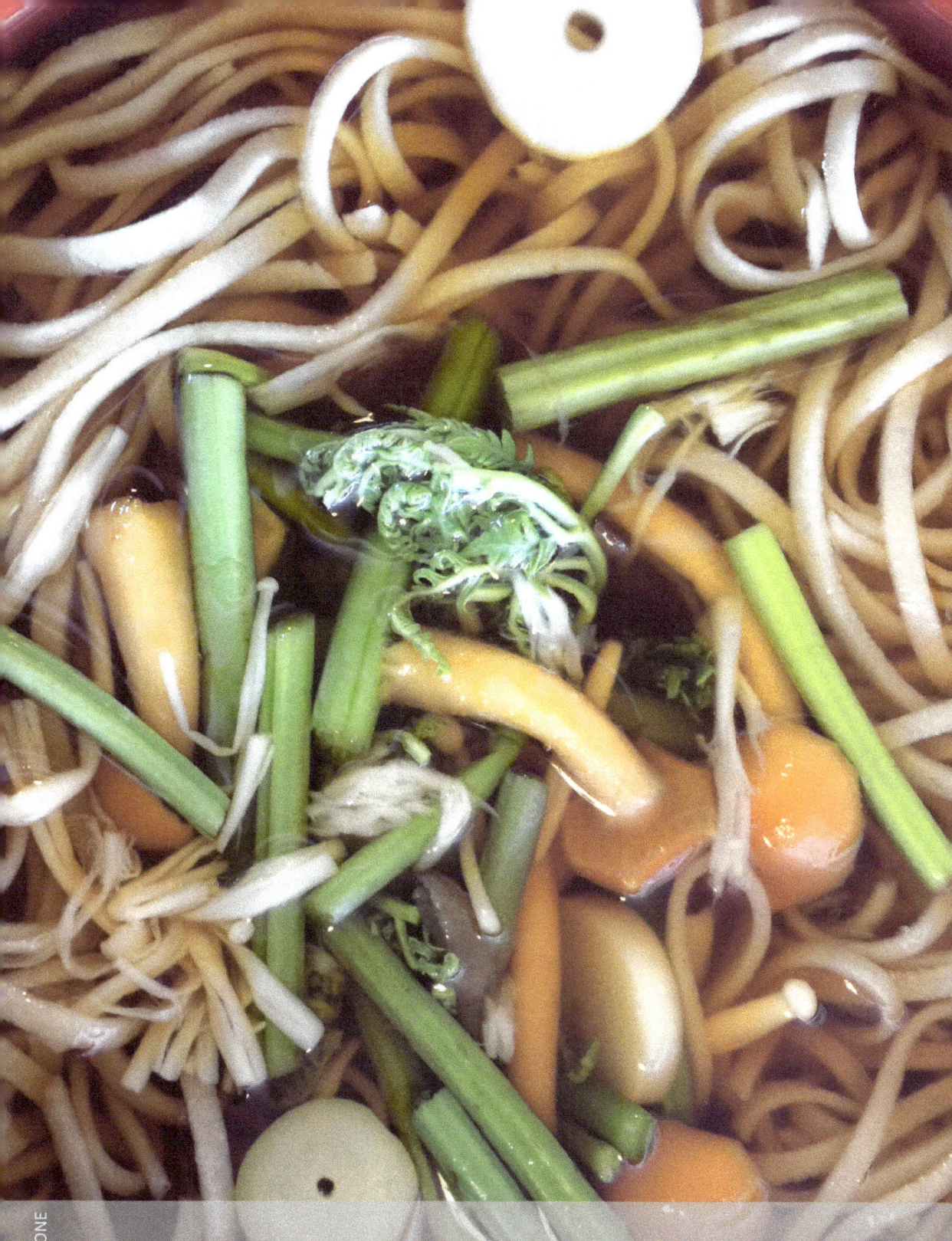

Gluten-free highlights in Honshu
Saitama, Takayama, Nikko, Nagano & Tazawako

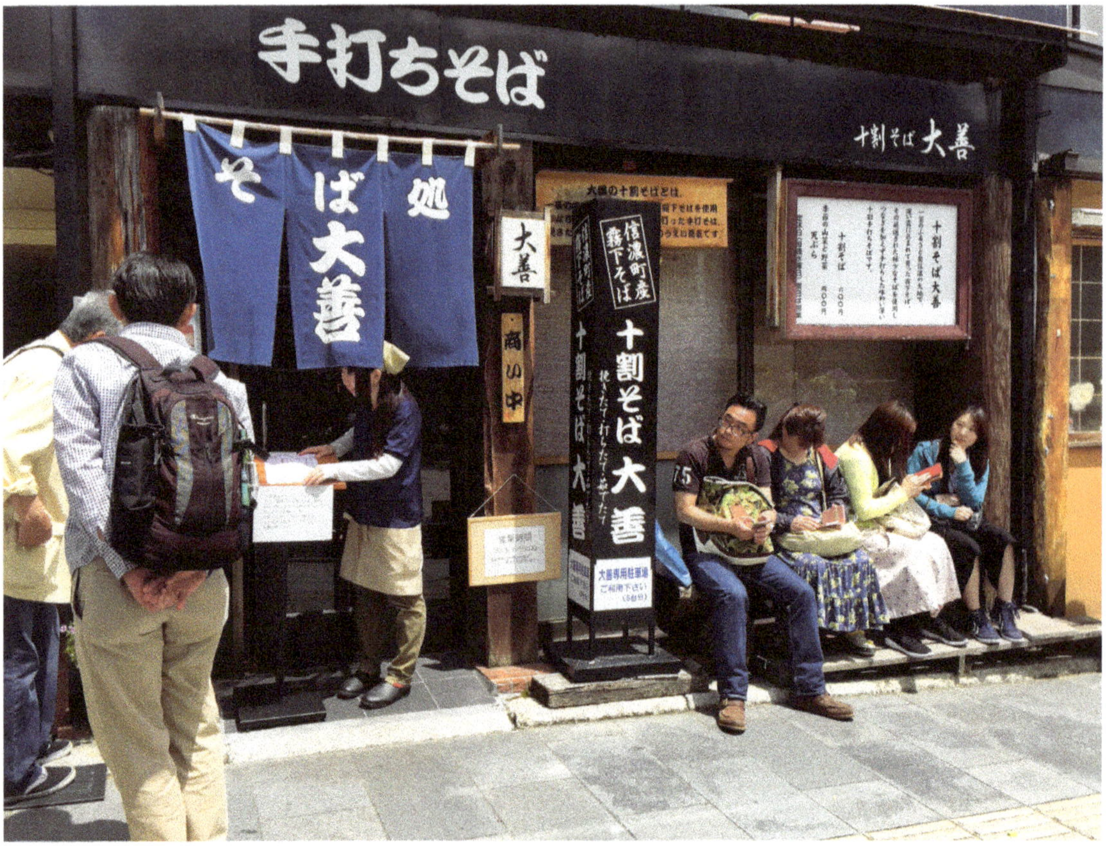

Above: Daizen 100% buckwheat soba restaurant, Nagano; Below Left: Part of meal at That Sounds Good Jazz Pension, Tazawako; Below Right Shabu-shabu restaurant, Saitama

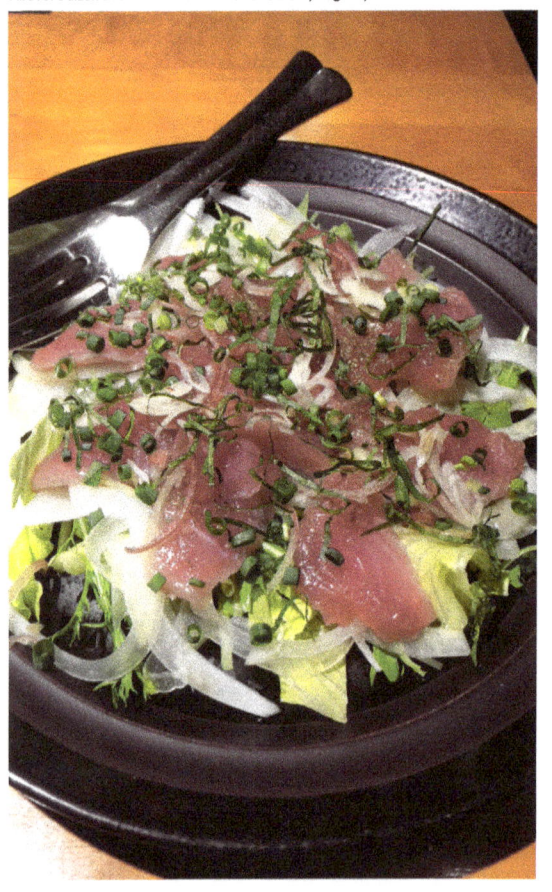
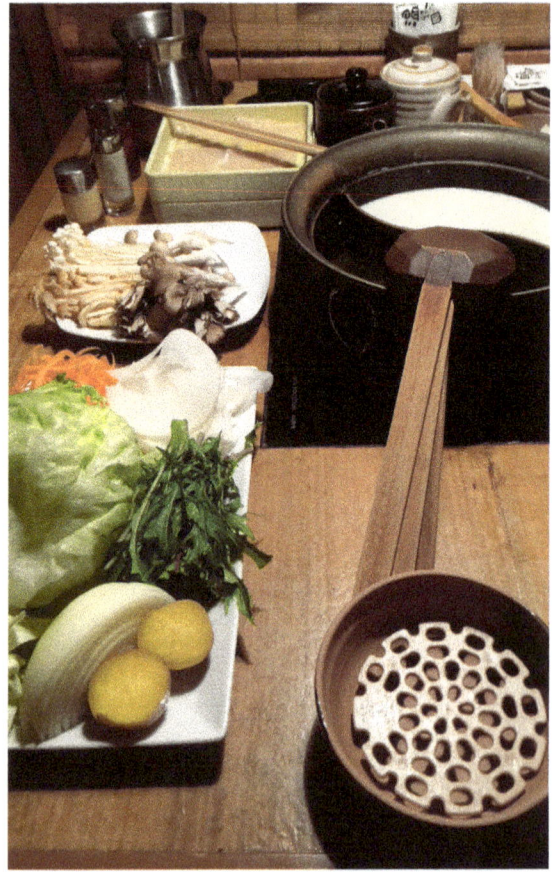

GLUTEN-FREE HIGHLIGHTS IN HONSHU: Saitama, Takayama, Nikko, Nagano, & Tazawako

Saitama

For much of our time in Tokyo we stayed in an Airbnb in Saitama, an outer suburb about an hour's train trip from the centre of the city. As with many Airbnbs, the joy is staying in neighbourhoods and getting a feel for the local life. We found some gems hidden away behind signs that we couldn't read. It's certainly worth checking out some of these places as you may get a pleasant surprise. One of the best discoveries was a shabu-shabu restaurant about half a kilometre from our house. It had an extensive menu both of ingredients — vegetables and/or various meats — and of broths. Many of the broth choices were gluten-free (e.g. soy milk) and you could have half one type of broth and half of another. They were ideal dishes for sharing and for socialising with friends whilst cooking your meal. As in most Japanese restaurants, the presentation was stunning. Another highlight in nearby Omiya was a sushi train restaurant in which the sushi was delivered by mini shinkansen trains — our visitors were very impressed!

Takayama

We had visitors who stayed with us for a short while in Saitama, after which we all headed off to Takayama in the mountains to the north. With them we discovered a really lovely restaurant quite close to the station that had a range of gluten-free meals. Until then we hadn't come across anywhere that had 100% buckwheat noodles on the menu. Buckwheat is grown in the mountains, which is no doubt why we hadn't seen any before. Unfortunately only a certain number of 100% buckwheat meals (both hot and cold dishes) were made each morning and they had run out by the time we arrived. Nevertheless, the dishes we had were very interesting and contained a selection of mountain vegetables that we hadn't come across before. After the visitors had left us, we returned another day at midday on the dot to sample the real soba, which were delicious. That day we also came across a cafe further up the hill which advertised gluten-free pancakes made with 100% rice flour, but, unfortunately, we were too full to try them out.

Nikko

The highlight of our stay in Nikko was our accommodation in the Suginamiki Youth Hostel. The hosts spoke excellent English and understood our need for gluten-free food. So we opted to have all our breakfasts and dinners with them. Since the place was some distance from the local station and surrounded by farms, we were treated to all the local specialities, including freshly picked edamame (soy beans), yuba (soymilk skin) and even chicken karaage (triple deep fried), made using rice flour.

Nagano

Nagano, famous for hosting the winter Olympics, is a mountain city where we found a restaurant called Daizen that served meals using 100% buckwheat soba noodles. Our meals were beautiful and featured soba along with a variety of mountain vegetables. However, be warned — the place is popular and there's always a queue outside.

Tazawako

It was an absolute delight to find a lovely pension out in the middle of the beautiful Japanese countryside on the eastern shore of Lake Tazawako. We returned to this part of the world because it had been so beautiful the last time we visited in winter — when we had relaxed in an outdoor onsen with snow falling around us. This time it was early summer and abuzz with insects visiting the green, vibrant plants.

The That Sounds Good Jazz Pension was not only a beautiful building, set in the forest, with rooms overlooking the lake (a 20 kilometre ride with bicycles supplied), but there was live music on some nights (unfortunately not during our stay) and our host prepared the most healthy and delicious meals you could imagine. She took on board our gluten-free requirement and cooked meals — from salads, to meat and egg dishes, to seafood including oysters, and home-made onigiri — that were not only appropriate but also very imaginative, using the very freshest of ingredients. Vegetables were the highlight through every meal, complementing the beautiful surroundings perfectly.

Photo Page 89: Hot-pot at Daizen 100% soba restaurant, Nagano

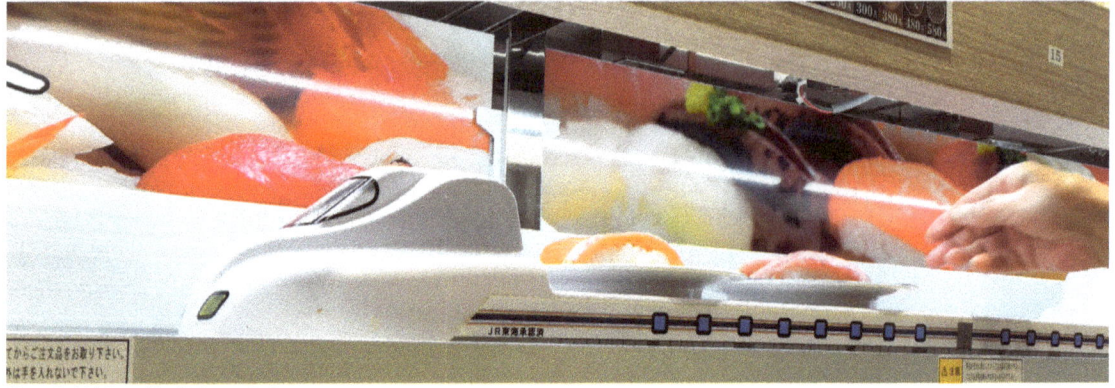
Above: Sushi delivered by shinkansen, Omiya

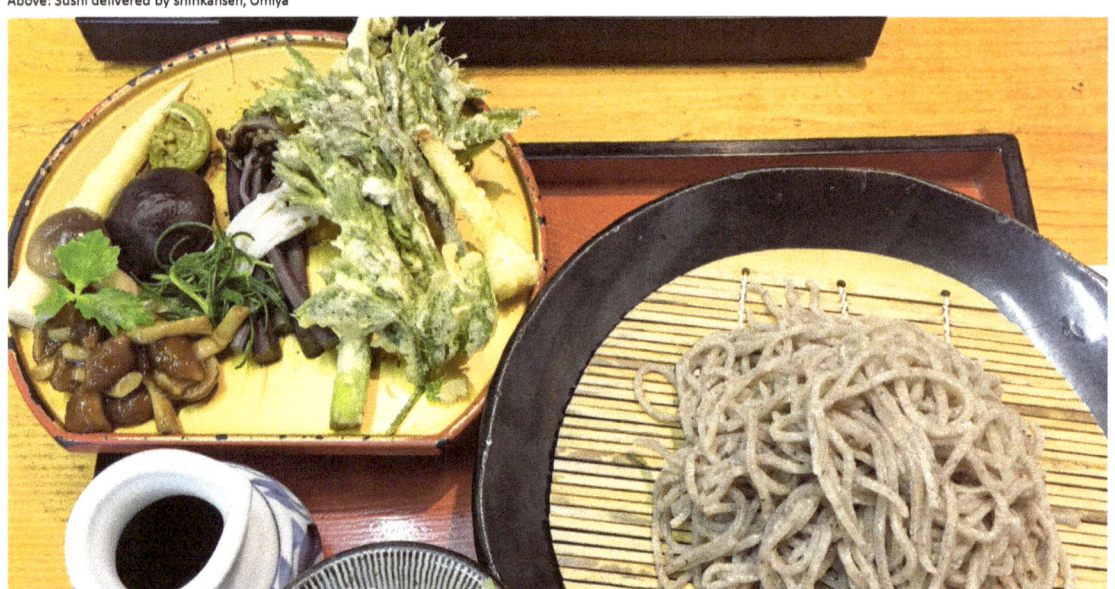
Above: Restaurant in Takayama with 100% buckwheat soba; Below: Gluten-free meal at Nikko Suginamiki Youth Hostel

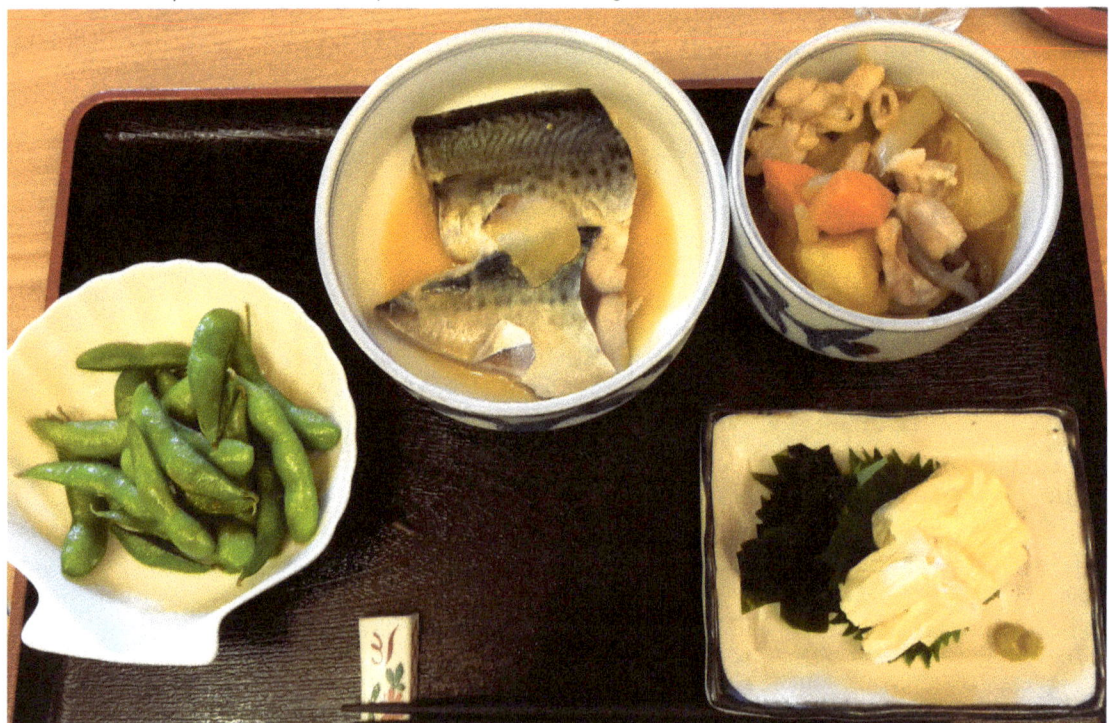

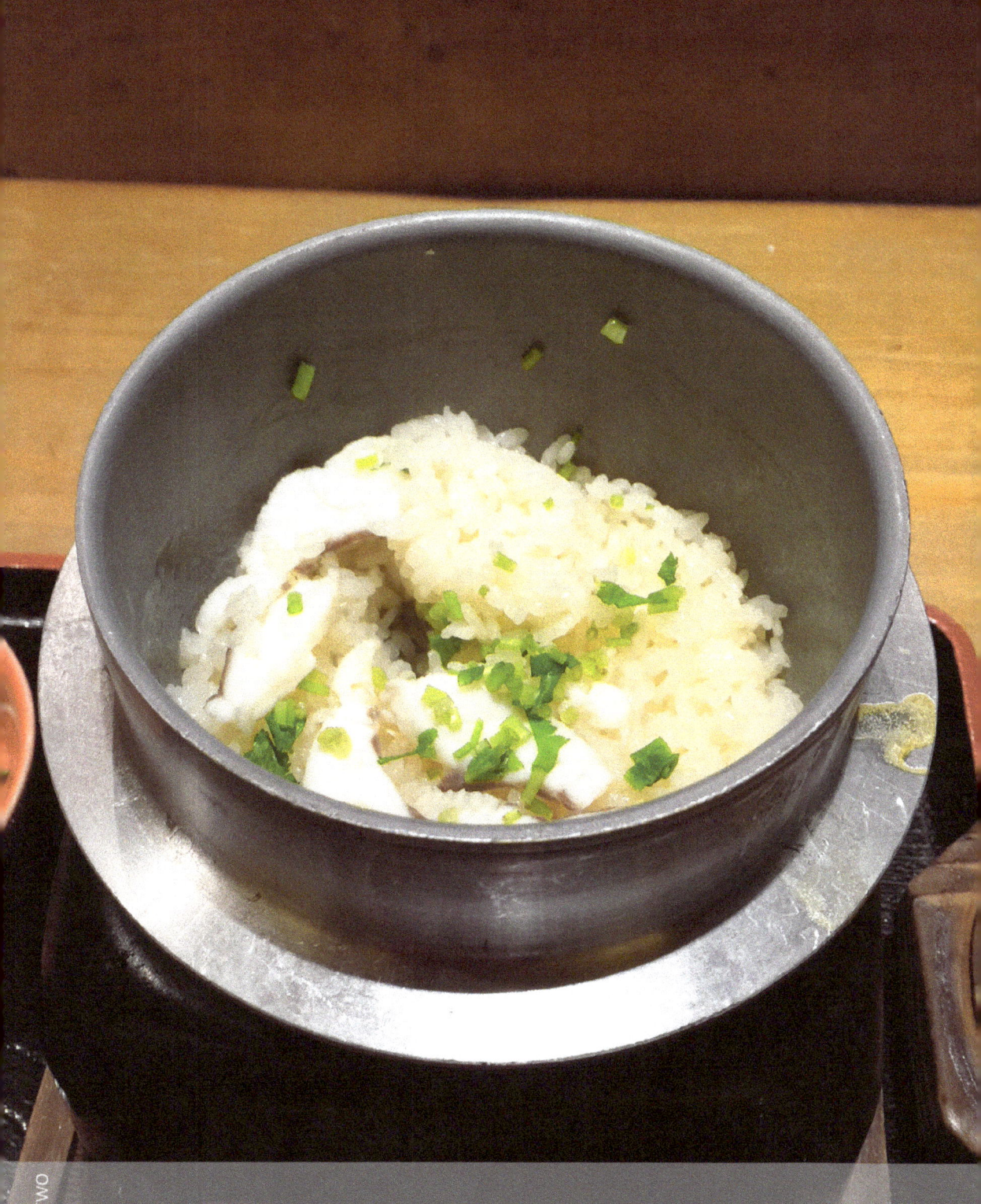

Gluten-free highlights in Shikoku
Naoshima, Matsuyama, Uchiko, Kochi & Sukumo

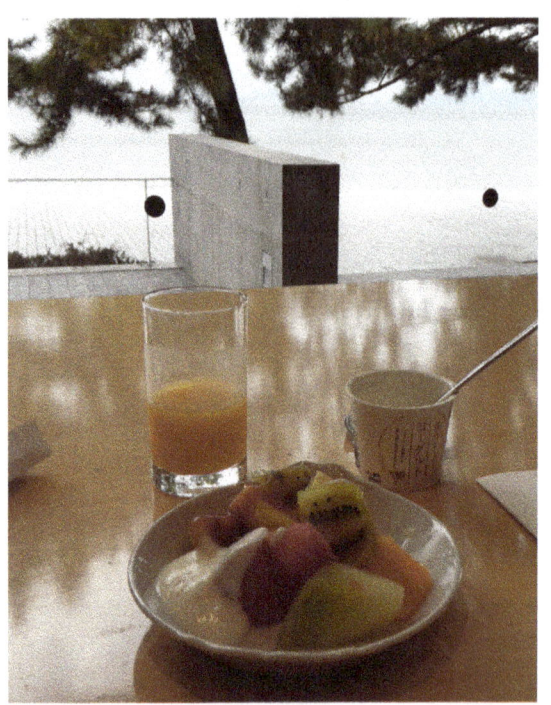
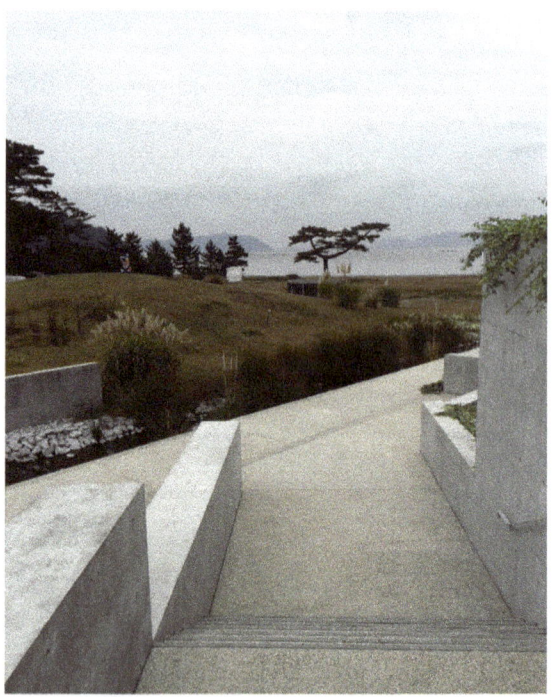

Above and Rows Below: Meals at Benesse House, Naoshima   Above: View from Benesse House, Naoshima

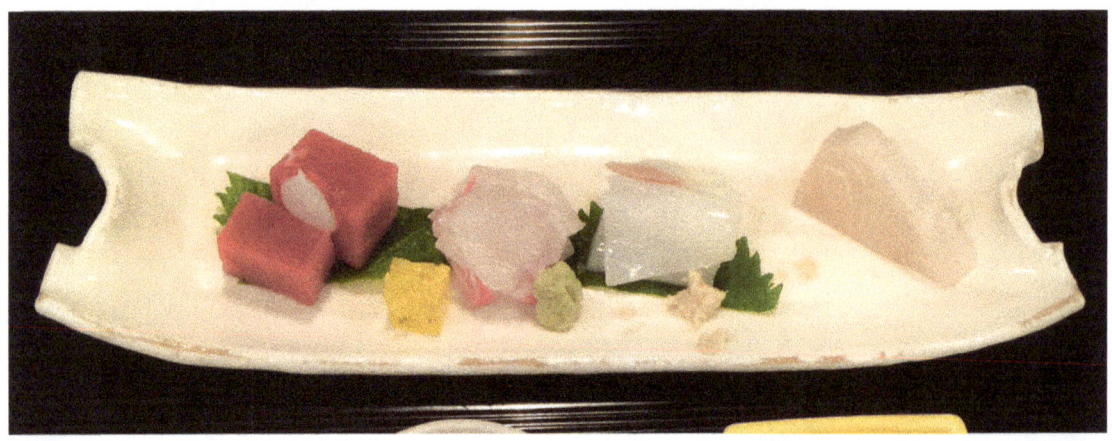
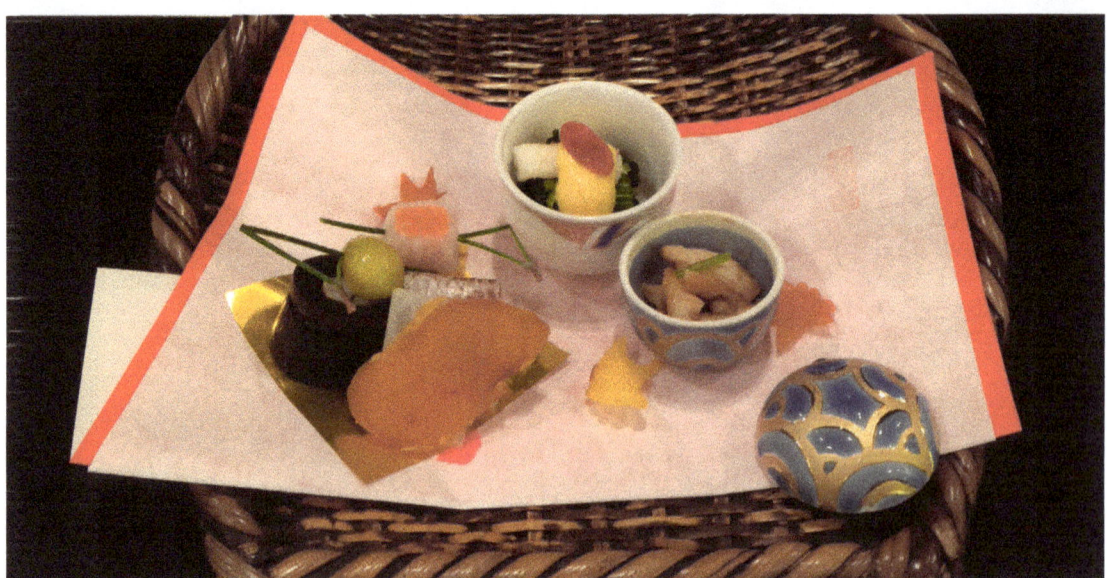

GLUTEN-FREE HIGHLIGHTS IN SHIKOKU: Naoshima, Matsuyama, Uchiko, Kochi & Sukumo

Naoshima

While there may have been many good restaurants in Takamatsu, we mostly cooked at home since we stayed in a lovely, trendy Airbnb that was some way out of town — just near the beautiful Ritsurin Garden which we visited several times. Our last night in Takamatsu coincided with the start of the Garden's nighttime illuminations at which we bought the most scrumptious fresh strawberry mochi (see Chapter 17). From Takamatsu we took a day trip to Teshima Island to visit the wonderful museum there and, when we finally left Takamatsu, it was on a ferry bound for Naoshima.

Both Teshima and Naoshima belong to the 'Art Islands', a group of islands on the Inland Sea that are mostly part of Shikoku and which host a three yearly Triennale event and display year-round an incredible world-renowned collection of modern art. On a friend's recommendation we had booked some time previously to stay at Benesse House on Naoshima. The accommodation was the most expensive of all the places we stayed at in Japan, but deemed necessary in order to see the artwork inside the hotel that isn't otherwise on public view. The place didn't disappoint and was certainly one of the highlights of our trip.

We had booked our breakfasts and dinners ahead of time and informed the hotel of our dietary requirements. On each of the two nights we enjoyed meals of delectable flavours, incredible quality and impeccible presentation. We each had our own menu printed on rice paper, a degustation of eight different courses: appetiser, soup, sashimi, fried dish, grilled dish, additional dish, a course of rice, miso soup and pickles, and a fruit or dessert course to finish (see Chapter 5). Needless to say, the service was outstanding too! There was a gorgeous water view from the breakfast restaurant and at dinner we were surrounded by beautiful pieces of modern art.

Matsuyama & Uchiko

While staying in Matsuyama, the capital of Shikoku, we found a lovely restaurant near the ropeway access to Matsuyama Castle that was open for lunch and served a rice lunch-set that featured the local dish of 'tail kameshi,' kettle-steamed rice with sea bream or snapper. Just near our accommodation at the historic area of Mitsu, we were also blessed with a range of great, cheap lunch places and we were also lucky enough to experience the Mitsu market open day event, which is only held a few times each year. But the highlight was a day trip to Uchiko, an hour south of Matsuyama, where there is an incredible amount to see and do, and where we found a small restaurant that served miso fish, another dish typical of the area. Everything in the lunch set was gluten-free and absolutely delicious.

Kochi

Right down on the south coast of Shikoku, lying almost midway between the spectacular eastern and western capes (Ashizuri and Muroto respectively) is the city of Kochi. The Kochi market is one of the biggest and probably the most interesting of all the markets in Japan. Here you can pick up a huge range of products, including many that are gluten-free. The range of seafood, vegetables and fruit is almost overwhelming and we found many nice things to snack on as we wandered around. There were plenty of mochi available, and seemingly every type of citrus fruit in existence — lemons, yuzu, mikan, tangerine, bankan, oranges and more. We also found a range of grilled sweet potato or yam slabs — interesting tastes and textures, though not our favourites. The market runs for 1.3 kilometres across several city blocks.

Sukumo

Mostly, we ate at home while in Sukumo, after once venturing out to a charcoal chicken restaurant. This was perhaps the most (or only) disappointing meal we had in Japan. Maybe it's an acquired taste, but the two different versions we tried were like eating charcoal. Nevertheless there are great local delicacies to be found in small shops as you're walking around or changing buses. While in the Sukumo area we sampled some of the really nice local takeaway bento boxes: sushi made with local vegetables ('inakazushi') and seared bonito sashimi ('katsuo no tataki'), which were both delicious.

Photo Page 93: Kettle steamed rice with sea bream, Matsuyama

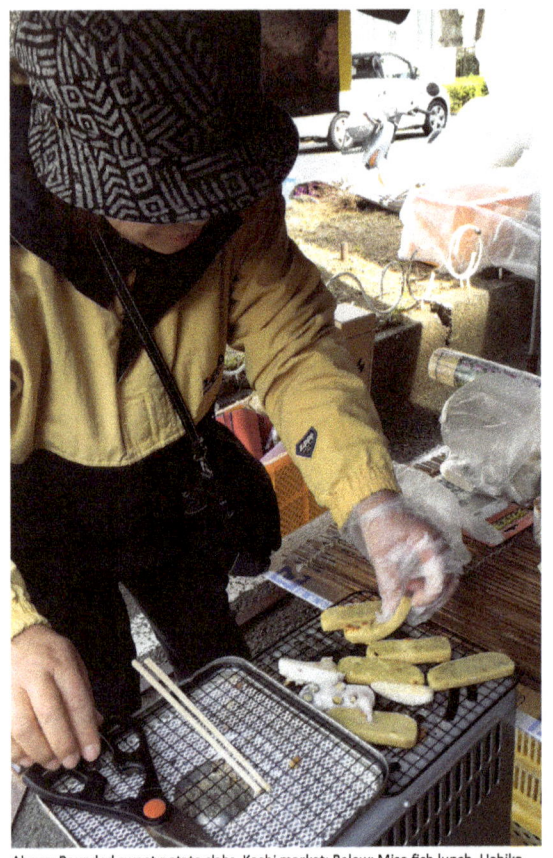

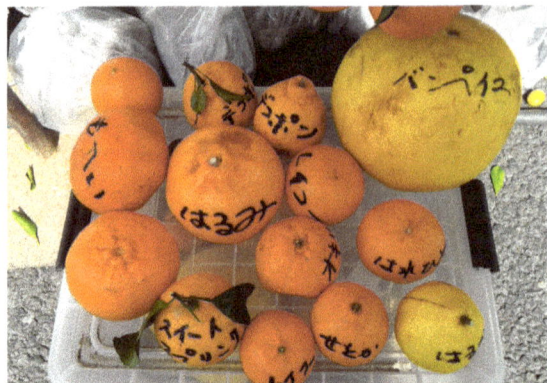

Above: Some of the various citrus varieties, Kochi Sunday market

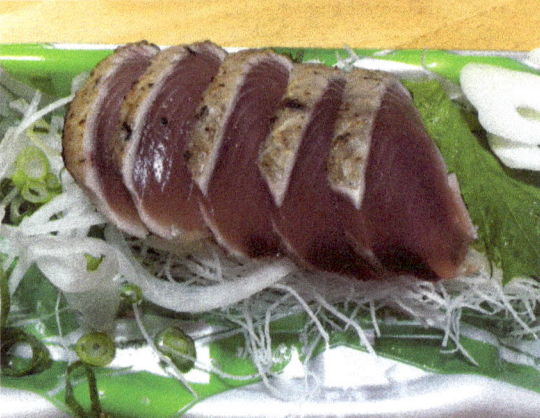

Above: Pounded sweet potato slabs, Kochi market; Below: Miso fish lunch, Uchiko

Above: Seared bonito sashimi, Sukumo

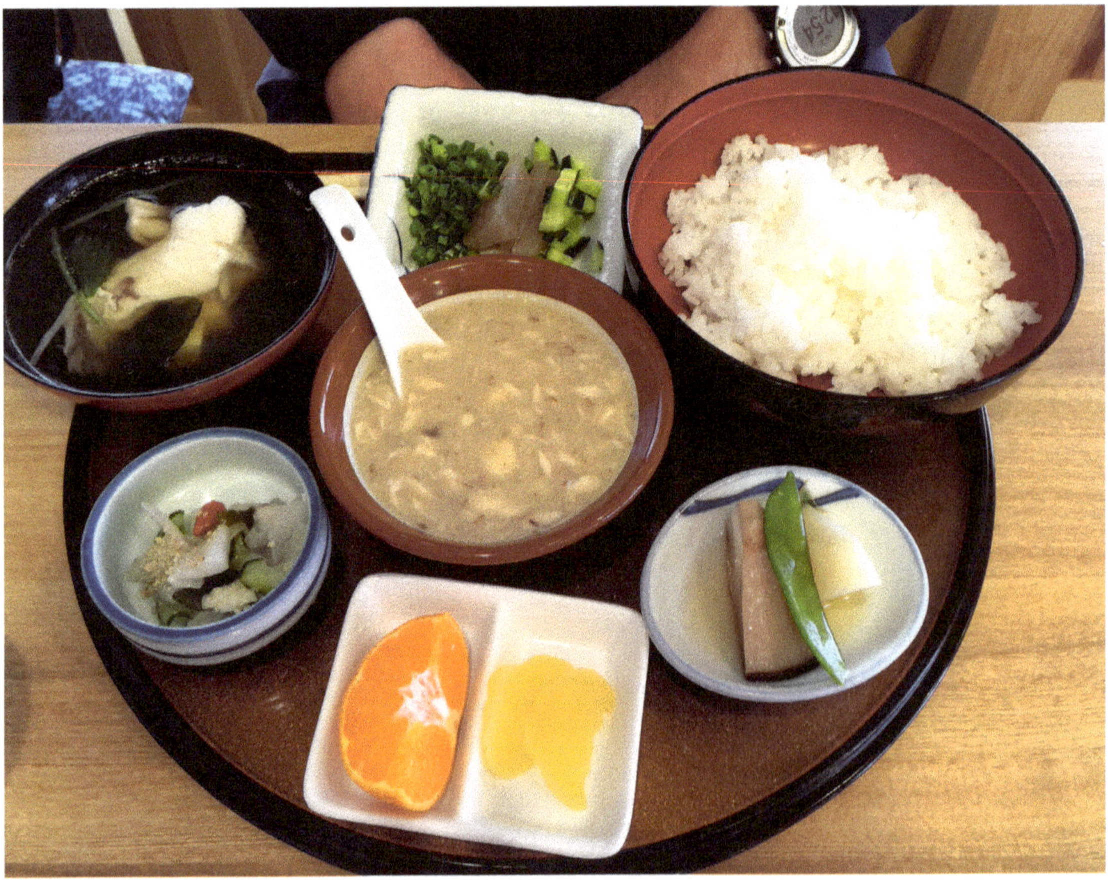

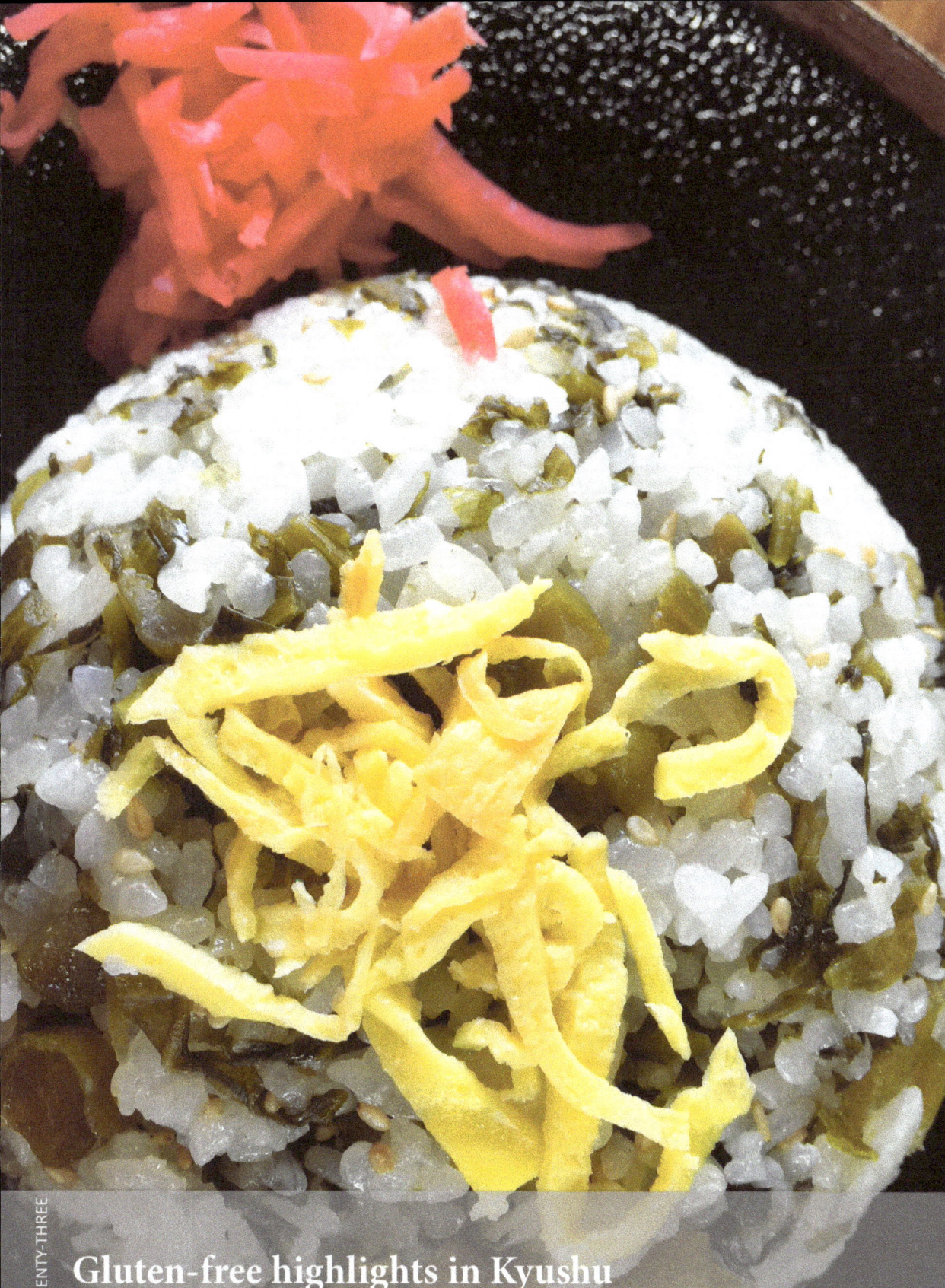

CHAPTER TWENTY-THREE

Gluten-free highlights in Kyushu
Fukuoka, Aso Town, Kagoshima & Yakushima

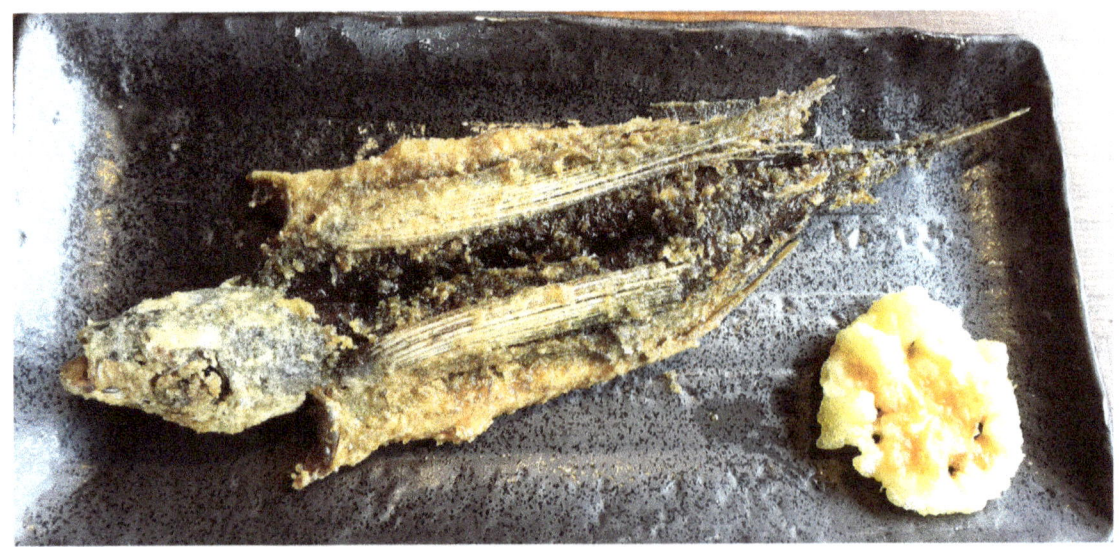
Above: Deep fried flying fish, Anbo, Yakushima; Below: Scallops at Sushi Isogai restaurant, Tenjin, Fukuoka

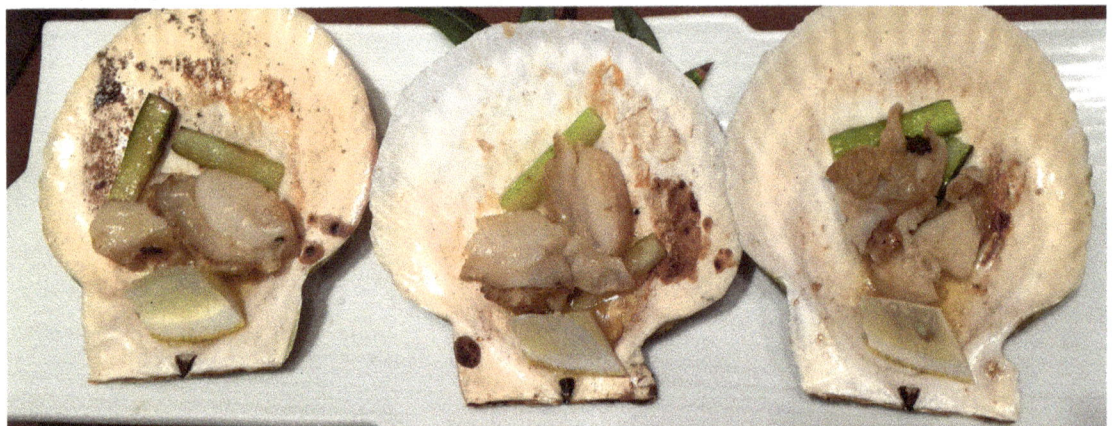
Below: Pickle rice and dumpling soup lunch set, Sanzoku Tabiji restaurant, Aso Town

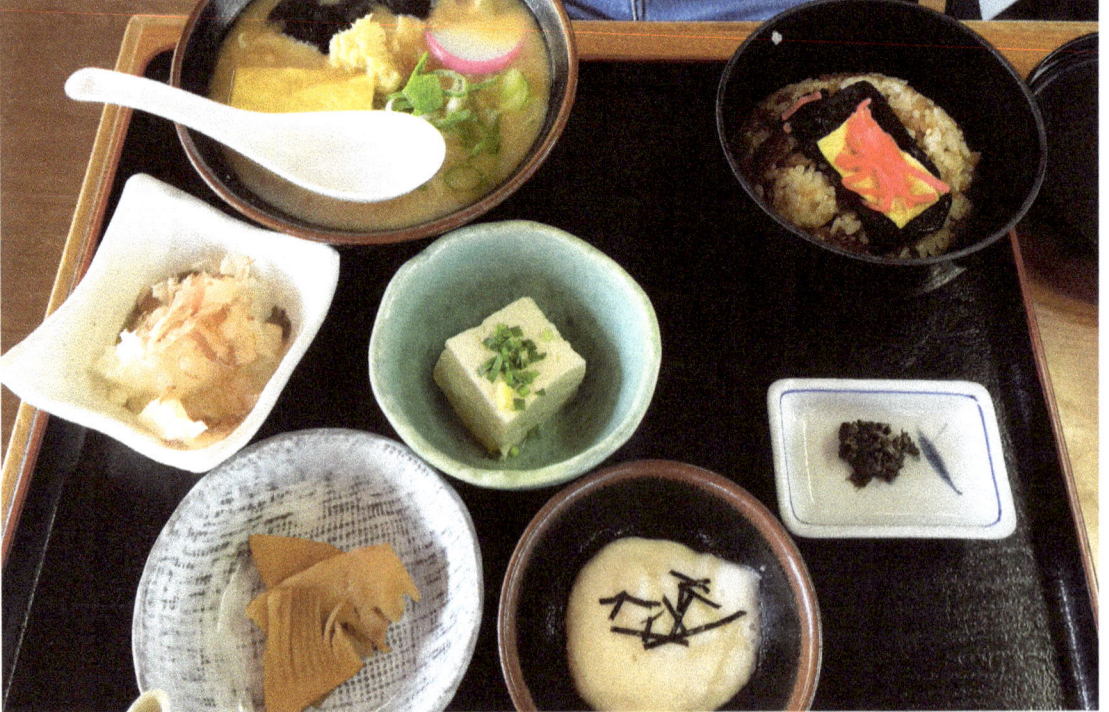

GLUTEN-FREE HIGHLIGHTS IN KYUSHU: Fukuoka, Aso Town, Kagoshima & Yakushima

Fukuoka

Fukuoka is a city divided into two parts by the river Naka. On one side is the newer centre of Tenjin, and on the other is Hakata, the older hub with port and Fukuoka's shinkansen station. You'll find a huge variety of restaurants in both parts of the city, though perhaps somewhat more in Tenjin. Look for quick lunch places around the stations or in the underground levels of department stores, as well as in the streets and alleys surrounding the stations. If you're after something a bit more classy, then you need to head to the top floors of buildings — usually the top two levels, with the topmost being the most pricey. On both floors you'll find a great mix of Japanese restaurants and other cuisines.

One of the highlights of the many weeks we spent in Fukuoka was a meal out with a friend at the upmarket Sushi Isogai restaurant in Tenjin. She was able to quiz the waiters and chef to determine which courses were or weren't gluten-free, so we were in safe hands to try a range of really delectible courses. As is the case everywhere you go in Japan, you basically get what you pay for, and in this case the slightly higher prices reflected exceptionally high quality and imaginative and beautiful presentation. The meal was truly exceptional.

Aso Town

Aso Town on the northern side of Mount Aso, the world's largest active volcano, boasts many volcano themed attractions. We went up the mountain on a very bleak day and after visiting the much over-rated Super Ring we walked back down in white-out conditions to reach the excellent Volcano Museum. Here we had a wonderful warming local vegetable hot-pot that was gluten-free. On another day we found the very good Sanzoku Tabiji restaurant for a set lunch featuring more local fare — pickle rice and vegetable dumpling soup (choice of wheat or rice). The entire ceiling of this restaurant was decorated with hanging ceramic dolls.

Kagoshima

We spent a night in Kagoshima prior to catching a plane to Okinawa where we were to spend a month — so as to be in the warmest part of Japan in winter. From the Remm Hotel in Kagoshima we wandered around the main restaurant area of the city in search of something for dinner but found nothing suitable for a coeliac and non-red meat eater. In one of the many brightly lit side streets we encountered a number of young men spruiking their restaurants and when we explained why they weren't getting our patronage, one of them kindly showed us to a fish restaurant on the fifth floor of a building a couple of blocks away.

The restaurant served awesome food! When we indicated we'd like some sort of fish, one of the chefs held up a large John Dory and we nodded 'yes, please!' He also promised some sashimi. We shared two of the most amazingly presented dishes we'd ever had. Everything (except the potato chips) had been scored to form intricately decorated pieces of art. The sashimi, some of which was slightly singed, curled to perfection, and was presented partly on a plate and partly within a box. The John Dory was expertly cooked with a coating of green herbs and its head and tail draped over opposite sides of a large plate.

Yakushima

Yakushima is an island located between Kagoshima and Okinawa, and is part of Kyushu. It's quite a unique island — you can drive arount the perimeter in half a day, yet in elevation it ranges from subtropical coral reefs at sea level to almost 2000 metres in the central mountains. It's a rugged environment and its mountains receive around ten metres of rain (and snow) per annum.

Little wonder then that Yakushima boasts some unusual dishes amongst its cuisine. The highlight for us was a visit to a lovely udon (noodle) restaurant by the sea in the town of Anbo, with our Airbnb hosts. The weather had turned foul and they kindly drove us around because they were more used to the driving conditions than we were. At the restaurant they explained our dietary requirements and the chef cooked up the Yakushima specialty of deep fried flying fish coated (specially for us) with potato flour instead of the usual wheat flour. The meal was superb!

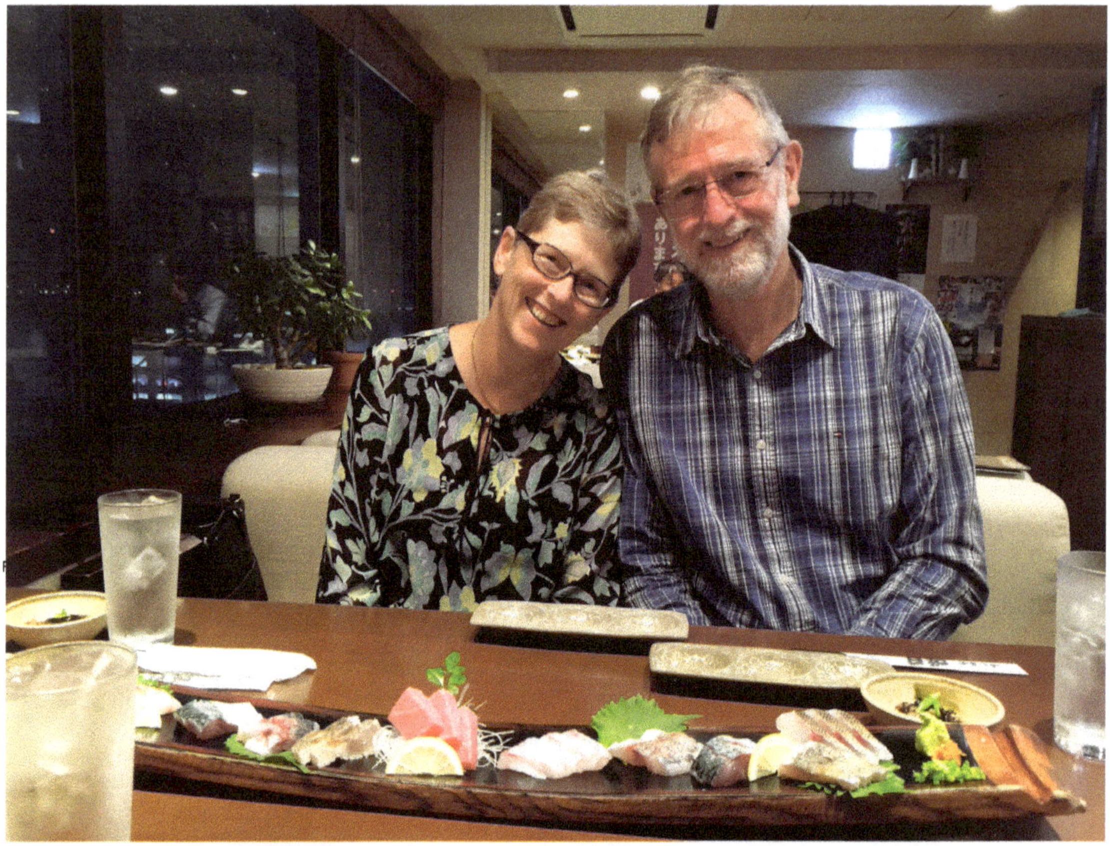

Above: Sushi Isogai restaurant, Tenjin, Fukuoka; Below: Ceramic dolls decorating ceiling, Sanzoku Tabiji restaurant, Aso Town

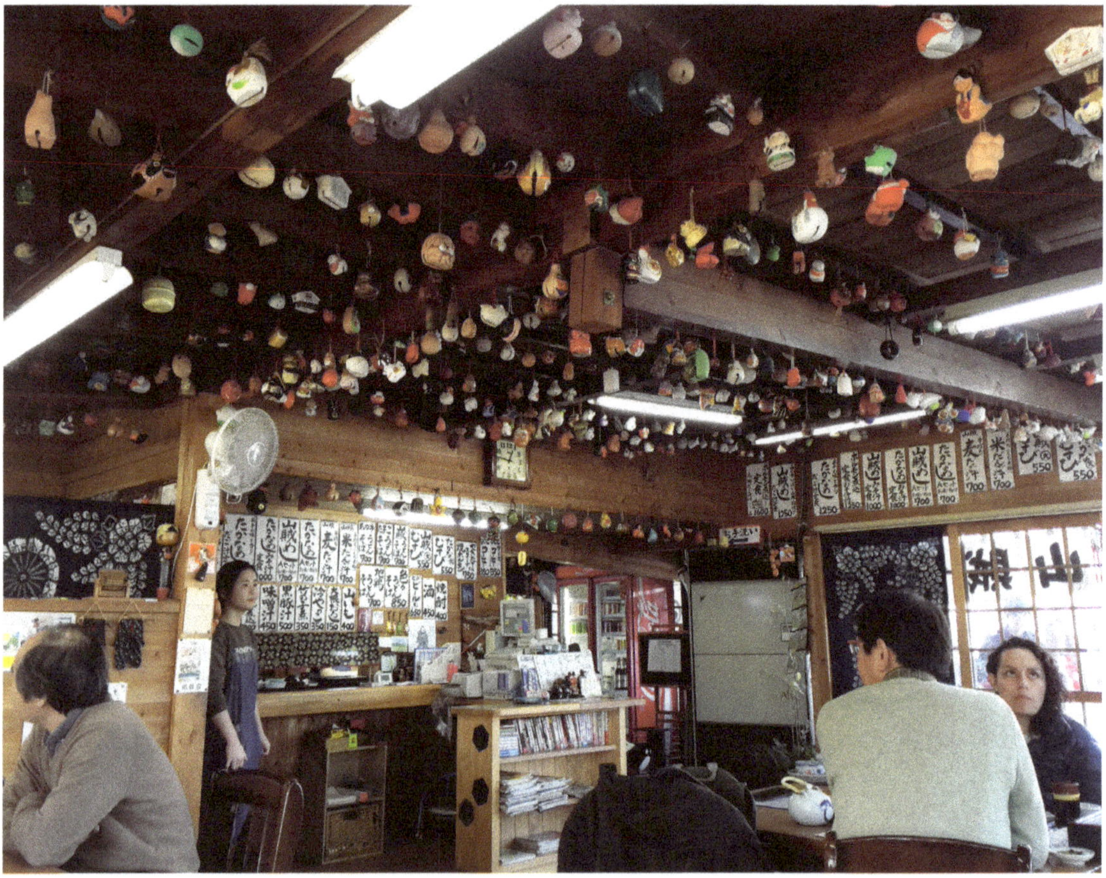

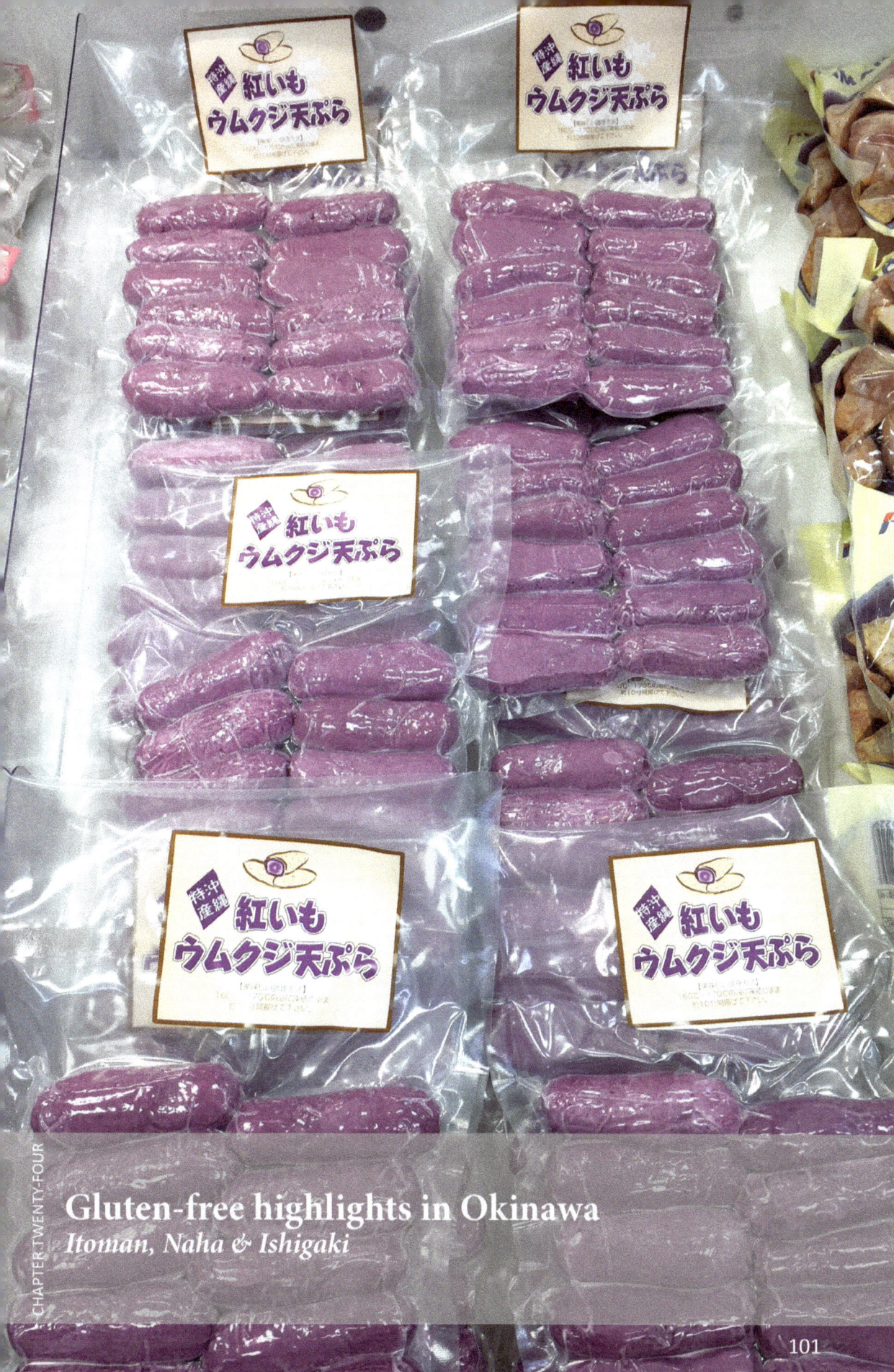

Gluten-free highlights in Okinawa
Itoman, Naha & Ishigaki

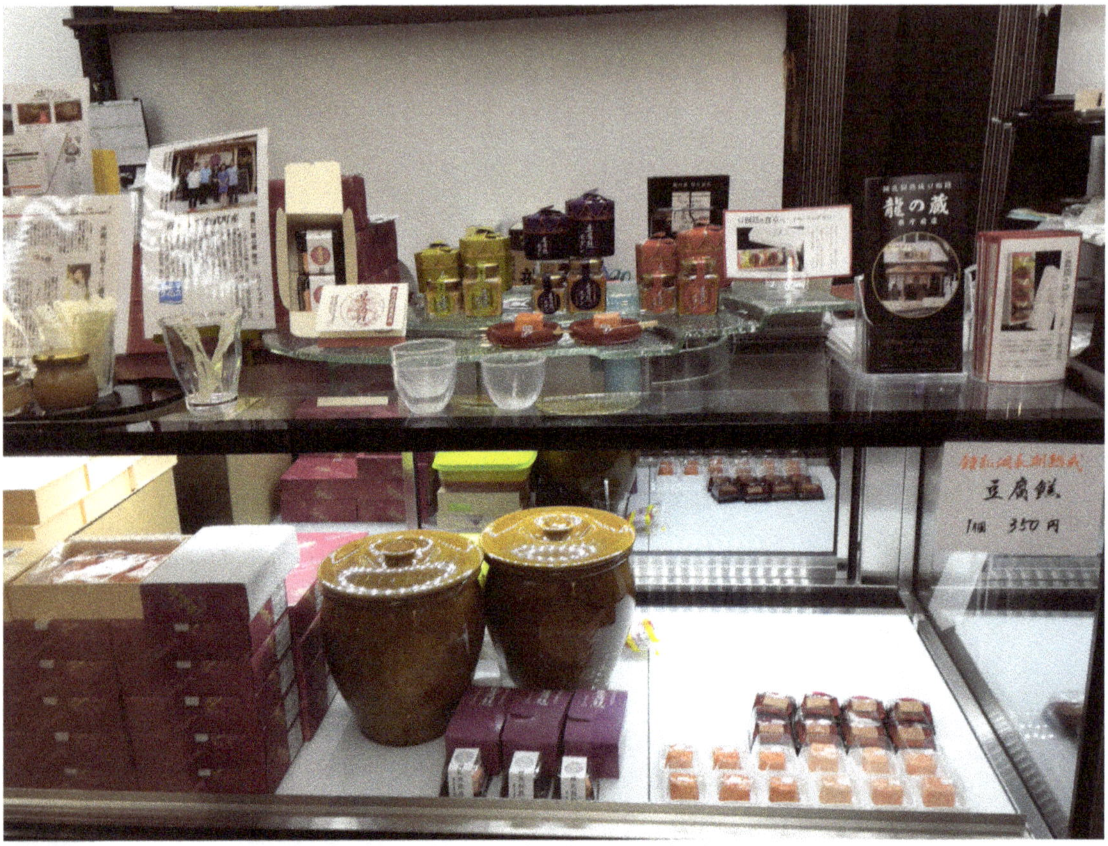

Above: Tofuyo shop, Naha, Okinawa; Below Left: Seafood at Itoman Fish Centre; Below Right: Taco rice, Naha, Okinawa

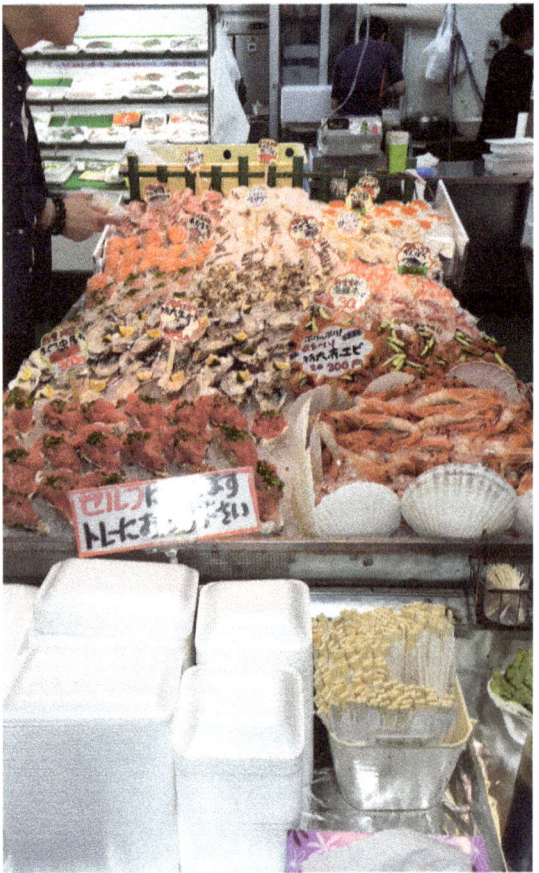

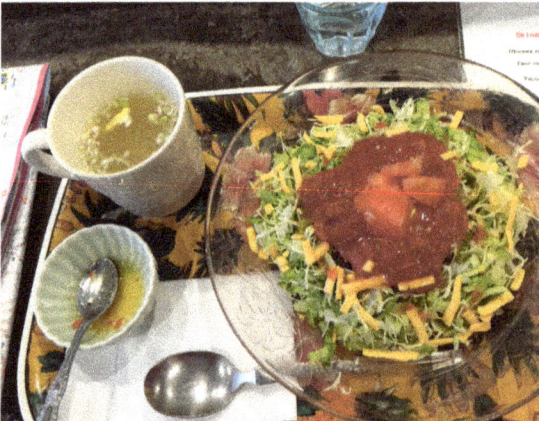

Below: Pickles at the Makishi Public Market, Naha, Okinawa

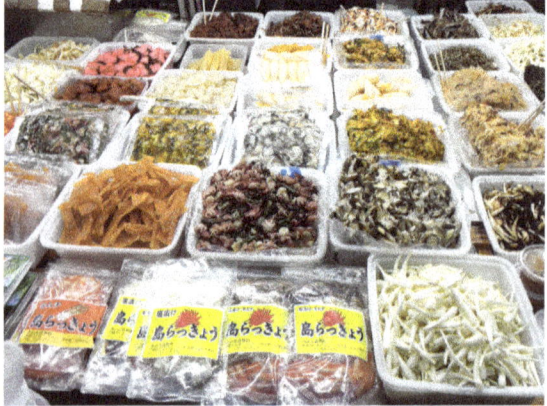

GLUTEN-FREE HIGHLIGHTS IN OKINAWA: Itoman, Naha & Ishigaki

Itoman

We rented an Airbnb in Itoman, about half an hour south of Naha, the capital of Okinawa. We rarely ate out at restaurants because the Growers' Market sold such beautiful fresh fruit and vegetables — including the purple, orange and yellow varieties that Okinawa is known for and which are so healthy due to their high content of anti-oxidants.

This Growers' Market also stocked a huge variety of snack foods and packaged foods, many of which were made from the purple vegetables, along with breads, cakes and fresh tofu (usually still warm). It was also the place to buy rice in bulk. Just outside the Growers' Market there were often flower stalls and sometimes a stall with fresh wakame seaweed.

Of course, much of the produce was gluten-free by its very nature, however there was a large stand of gluten-free packaged products labelled in English as well as Japanese — including gluten-free soy sauce and various types of noodles such as ramen, spaghetti and fettucinne.

Next door to the Growers' Market was the Itoman Fish Centre, which sold fresh seafood to take home and cook, along with seafood to eat at their tables — soups, lobsters cooked with miso, scallops, and more. There were more seafood and produce sellers at the port, which was slightly closer to home. As well, we had an excellent AAA (SanA) Shopping Centre nearby.

We tried the restaurant attached to the AAA supermarket for a lunch on almost our last day in Itoman, only to discover that they served a number of gluten-free dishes, including a really good shabu-shabu, in which the meat and vegetables were cooked in a soy milk broth. This became a new highlight that we wished we'd discovered much earlier on! Another huge highlight in Itoman was to be able to share the New Year's Eve celebrations with our Airbnb host's family, with shared finger food that we could pick and choose from. It was a real privilage to be invited, and especially to accompany the family for prayers (and awamori!) at the local shrine after midnight.

Naha

A real highlight in Naha is the tofuyo shop. Tofyu is aged tofu fermented in awamori (strong distilled sake). It's so rich that it's eaten only in tiny quantities, usually as an accompaniment to alcoholic beverages such as awamori, shochu or sake. The taste is exquisite and not unlike a rich blue cheese.

If you're interested in local fare, two other highlights (if you can call them that!) in Naha are taco rice (meat and salad sitting on rice instead of being in a taco or tortilla shell) and spam (tinned cooked pork). Dishes incorporating spam are widespread and very popular in Okinawa, where you can buy at least half a dozen different varieties in the supermarket. This particular food is a hangover of the American influence during the Second World War. While spam dishes might be a highlight for some, they definitely weren't for us, despite all spam varieties being gluten-free.

Ishigaki

We spent a week on Ishigaki Island, one of the Yaeyama Islands in the far south of Japan. The further south you travel in Japan, the more tropical fruits you encounter — such as the tropical fruit and sugar cane juice drinks at the Yonehara Palm Grove (see Chapter 19).

But the real highlight on Ishigaki was a small restaurant we stumbled across and checked out during the day with the intention of coming back for dinner. Unfortunately (!!) the spam with avocado was only on the lunchtime menu, so we had to settle for a different selection at dinnertime. We chose only gluten-free dishes from the menu (with the manager's help) and ended up with some very unusual dishes, such as soft deep fried tofu, barbecued leeks, potatoes with squid and a chicken dish — all of which were very nice.

Budget Travel in Japan

Budget Travel in Japan is the title of my accompanying book, in which you can read about our adventures week-by-week during our year in Japan. It's full of all the travel photos I didn't have room to include in this book!

Photo Page 101: Purple sweet potatoes at Growers' Market, Itoman, Okinawa

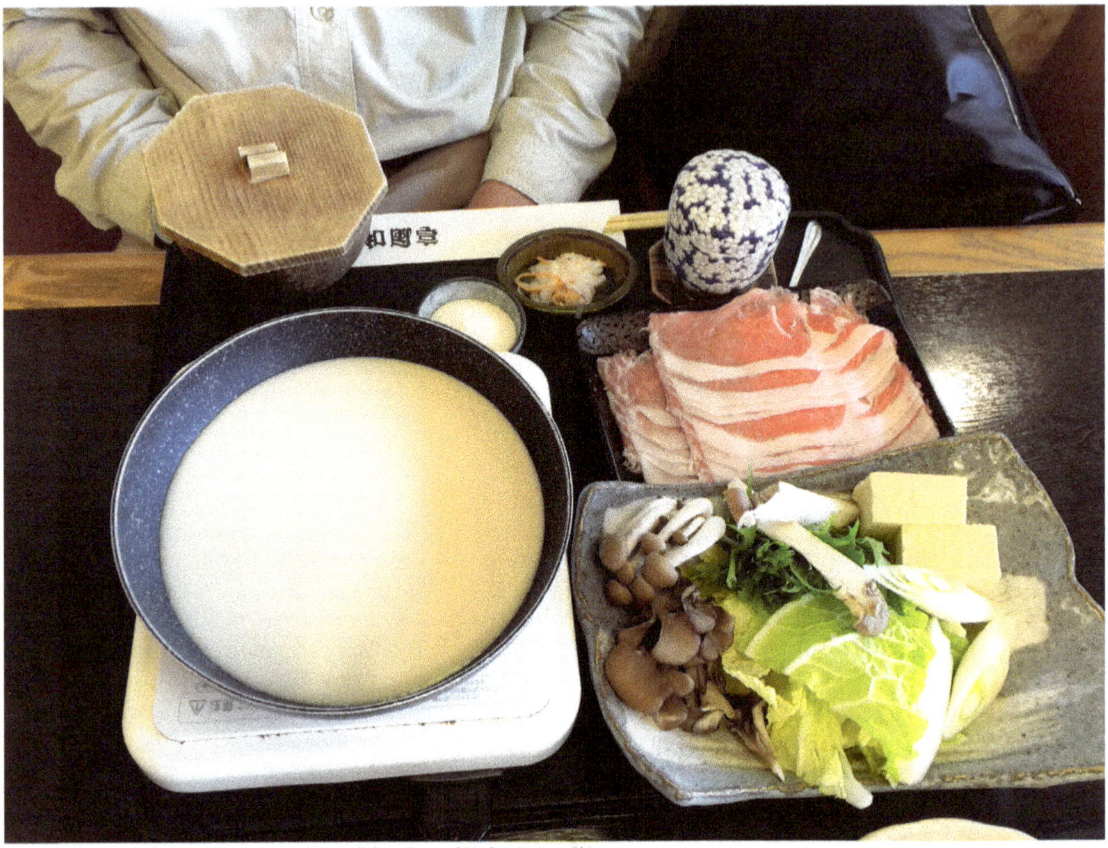

Above: Soy milk shabu-shabu lunch at Itoman, Okinawa; Below: Growers' Market, Itoman, Okinawa

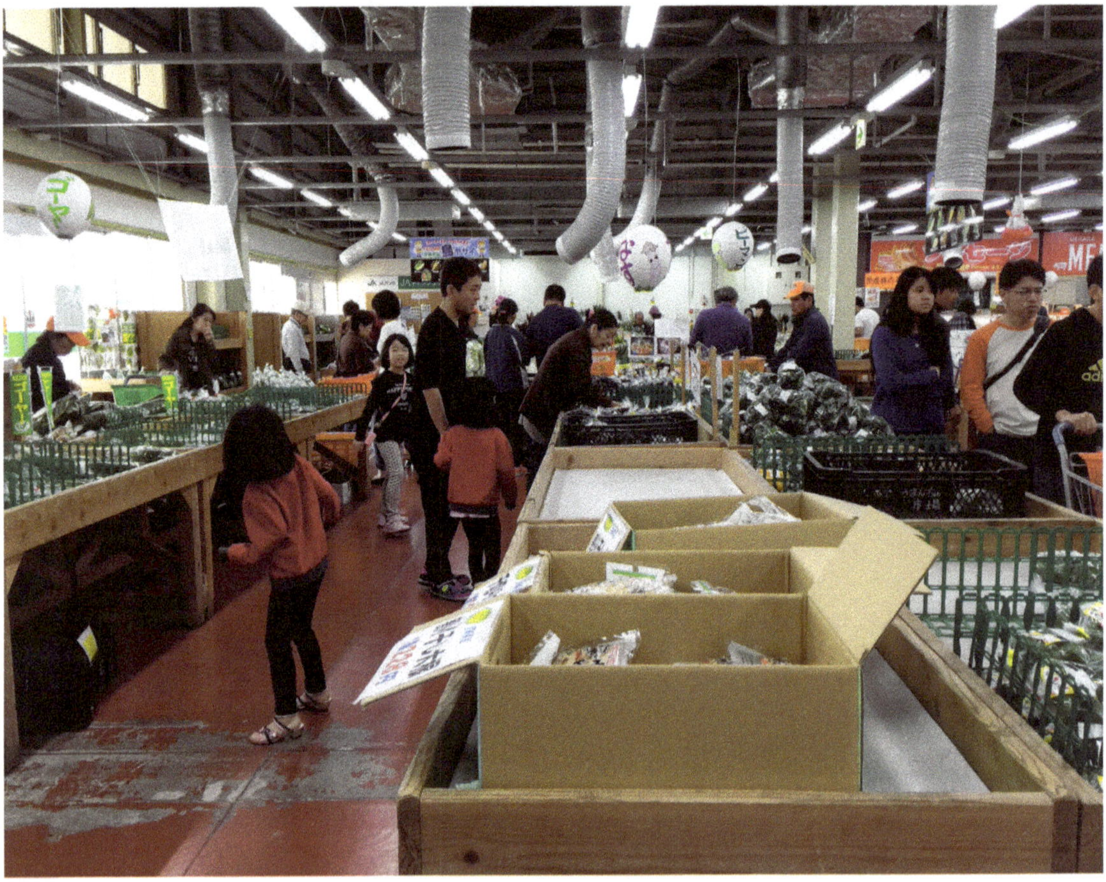

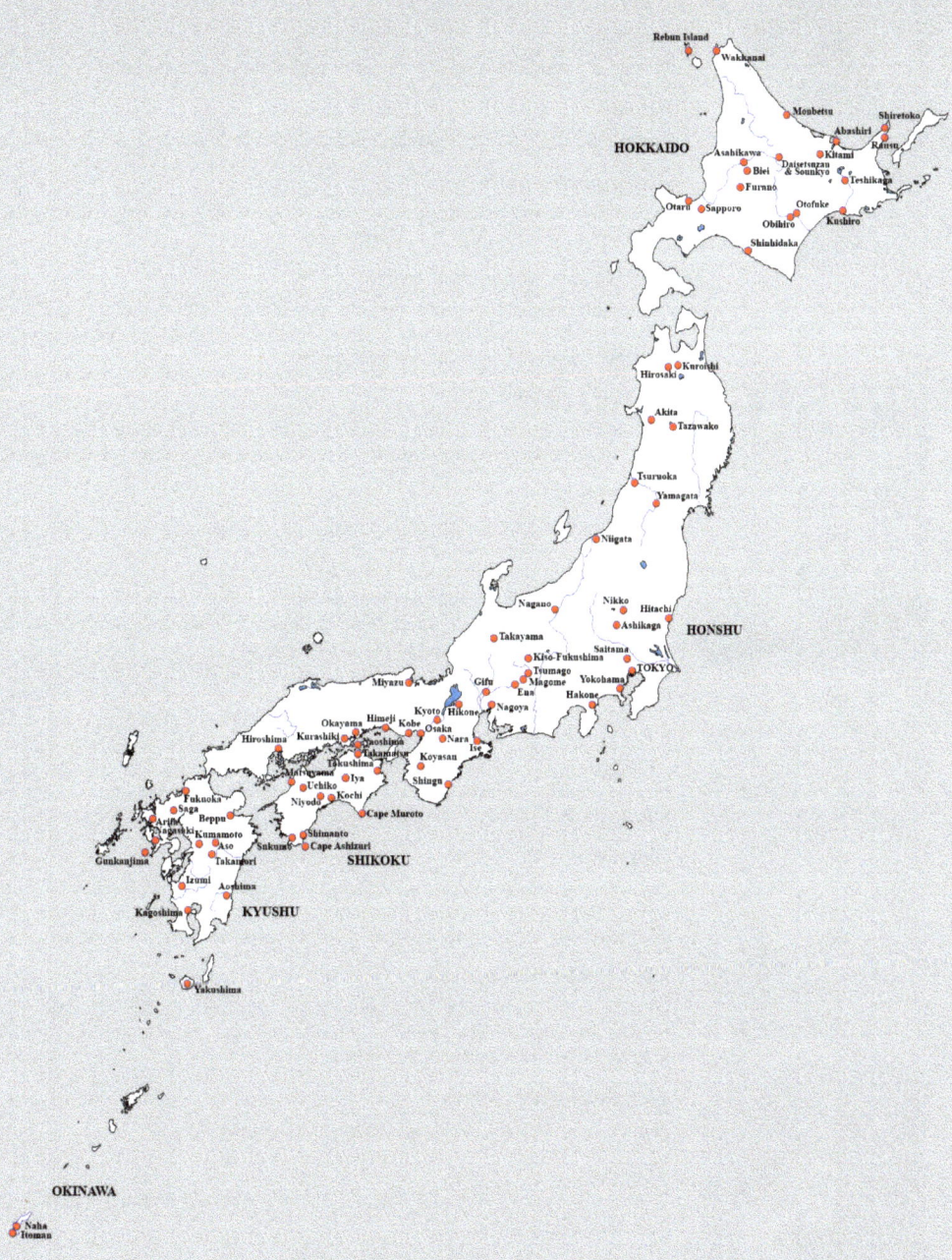

Map showing main locations mentioned in text

PRACTICAL TIPS & ADVICE

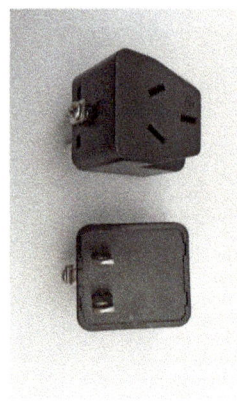

Adaptors
Voltage in Japan is 100V and you'll need a plug with two straight pins.

Alcohol
Beer is similar in price to Australia; spirits, wines, sake and shochu are cheaper than in Australia.

Booking accommodation
Accommodation websites such as booking.com are reliable and easy to use. All Airbnbs listed in Japan have to be accredited and so are reliable.

Booking entertainment or sports
Use vending machines at convenience stores where the staff will be happy to help you. Book seats for sumo tournaments through the English online website, as soon as bookings open; chair seating is available in the upper rows but sells out quickly.

Booking transport
Look up train timetables online or search for routes in Google Maps. Make a list of the trains you want to catch and show the list at a Japan Rail ticket counter where they will issue the tickets.

Budgeting
Our budget was $300 per day for two people, all inclusive of accommodation, transport and meals.

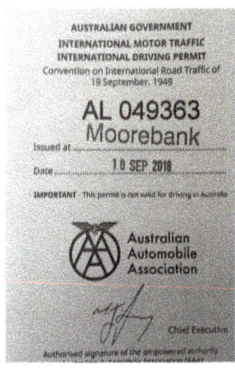

Clothes
Pack light and choose clothing appropriate for the season. Layers of clothing are best if moving in and out of heated public transport, stores or houses. Clothes are quite expensive to buy in Japan, and might not be available in larger sizes. Take your own.

Currency & credit cards
The Japanese currency is the yen. Cash is still the preferred payment method, and big bills are usually accepted, although you'll need coins for storage lockers and buses generally do not accept bills above 1000 yen. Cash is best for entrance fees at tourist venues, small restaurants and shops. Credit cards are usually accepted in hotels, department stores, larger restaurants, convenience stores and supermarkets. IC cards, used mainly for transport, can also be used for payment in many places.

Driving
Japanese drive on the left hand side, though they usually walk on the right hand side. If you intend to drive in Japan, you will need an International Driver's Licence. If you hire a car in Japan, make sure you request an English language 'navi'. Car hire costs are similar to Australia.

Earthquakes & tsunamis
Download the 'Safety tips' application to receive early warnings and advisories of disasters and weather warnings. Available in many different languages. Register with the Australian Department of Foreign Affairs (or equivalent) before leaving.

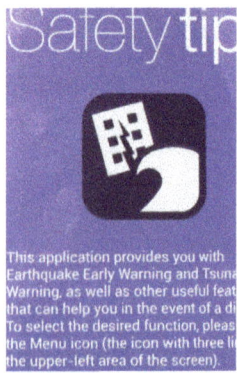

Emergency phone numbers
Phone 119 for fire and ambulance. Phone 110 for police.

Etiquette
There are many rules of etiquette that foreign visitors should be aware of before visiting Japan. There is a wealth of information online.

Events
There are many events, festivals and public holidays in Japan, so it's a good idea to check them out online. It may be hard to find accommodation during peaks of cherry blossom and autumn foliage, or in Golden Week or O-Bon. On the other hand you may wish to plan your visit around these events.

Garbage & recycling
Most accommodation other than hotels will require you to separate your garbage into three, or up to fourteen, different categories for recycling — such as paper/cardboard, PET bottles, glass, aluminium.

Internet, wi-fi, data
Most types of accommodation provide wi-fi or mobile wi-fi. You can rent your own mobile wi-fi by booking online and picking up a device at the airport on arrival. Handy for using Google Maps and Google Translate while on the move.

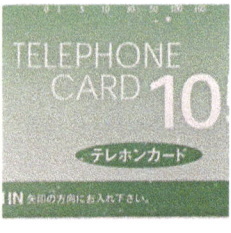

Japan Rail Passes
Japan Rail Passes make train travel very economical if you are doing a lot of travelling in a short time,

especially if you're using shinkansens. Available as 7-day, 14-day or 21-day options, ordinary class or green (first) class. Buy online at least seven days before you leave. Also available at Tokyo Station. Major stations have a ticket counter especially for Rail Pass bookings, with English-speaking staff.

Language
Japanese is a very difficult language to learn. However, railway station signage includes names in romaji (English alphabet) for previous, current and next stops. Google Translate is helpful, but not perfect, especially for reading labels.

Laundry
Laundromats (coin laundries) are abundant in Japan. They have a wide range of washers, dryers, and also change machines. Note that some machines add the laundry powder automatically. Most types of accommodation, including hotels, have coin-operated washers and dryers available for guests to use.

Luggage
Travel light, there's not a lot of room for large bags on trains and few very large storage lockers at stations. The luggage forwarding system for sending luggage from one hotel to the next is excellent.

Medical & hospitals
If you want to take more than a month's worth of medicines into Japan, you will need to fill out a 'yakkan shoumei' (medicine importation) form, have it approved by email before you leave, and present it at immigration on the way in. Check online for banned drugs such as pseudoephedrine.

The Japanese medical system doesn't work by referrals from general practitioners. If you are unwell, it's best to go to a large hospital (with many different departments) or directly to the relevant specialist clinic (e.g. ear-nose and throat, orthopedic, etc.). Without a Japanese health card you will have to pay upfront. However, the costs are reasonable and the system is efficient.

The clinic or hospital will prescribe medicines and the pharmacy will usually get an English speaker on the phone to check your medical history and explain dosages. You should be able to claim on your travel insurance.

Mobile phones & laptops
Use your own mobile phone but be careful of roaming charges. Or select a plan that charges a flat fee for 24 hours if activated. Or rent a phone. SIM cards are usually for data only, not voice calls. Phone cards for public phones are available at convenience stores.

Onsens
Onsens or spa baths are places to relax. They may be indoor or outdoor or a mixture of both. They are usually separate for men and women, and strict procedures and etiquette must be observed (check online). Most onsens don't accept visitors with tattoos due to an old association with organised crime.

Seniors discounts
In Japan, older people qualify as Seniors at either 65 or 70 years of age, depending on the place. Usually the discounts only apply to residents, and sometimes only to residents of the immediate local government area. Some major attractions offer discounts for overseas tourists with appropriate passports.

Tea, coffee, hot chocolate
Plenty of options are available as hot and cold drinks from vending machines and convenience stores. Tea and coffee are usually available in either black or white, and most are sweetened. However you'll find other styles of coffee like cappucinos and lattes at cafes like Starbucks. Instant and drip coffee bags are available from supermarkets.

Transport cards
IC cards, such Suica, Nimoca and Icoca, are stored-value cards used primarily for public transport. Most cards, no matter where they are purchased, can be used Japan-wide.

Visas
You won't need to obtain a visa before you travel to Japan, as 90-day tourist visas are issued upon arrival. If you intend to stay longer, the easiest option is to leave the country (e.g. go to South Korea) and return a short time later. Six-month sightseeing visas are available but require a lot of paperwork. They can be renewed for a further six months while in Japan, within three months of the expiry date.

Water
Tap water is safe to drink throughout Japan.

Weather
Japan experiences typhoons from July to October, especially in August and September. Expect snow in winter as far south as Kyushu, with rail and road closures further north.

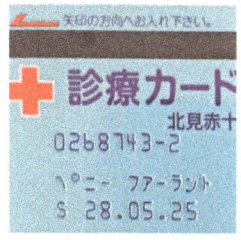
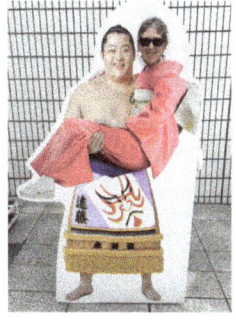
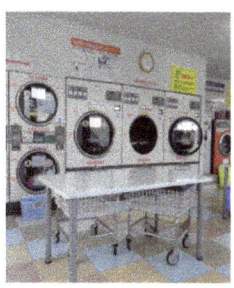
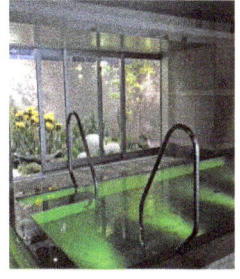
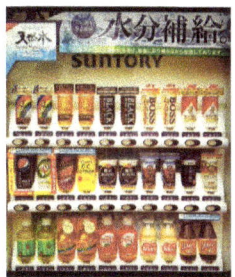
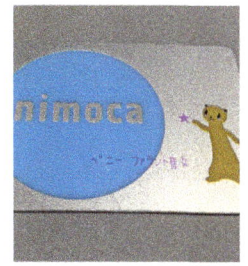

Index

A

Accommodation 15, 19, 31, 59, 106
    Airbnbs 3, 15, 31, 51, 55, 83, 91, 95, 99, 103, 106
    Apartment 15, 55
    Guest Houses 87
        Guest House Yasumizaka 30
        Yasumizaka Guest House 87
    Hostels 3, 15, 31
        Grids Hotel and Hostel 31, 54
        K's House Hostel 15, 31
    Hotels 3, 15, 27, 28, 31, 59, 78, 106
        Benesse House 26, 27, 94, 95
        Hotel Kinoe Sou 27, 28
        Remm Hotel 99
        Shuho Royal Hotel Shuhokan 27
        Touakarino Yado Rausu Daiichi Hotel 27
        Tswano Hotel 27
    Pensions 3, 31
        Pension Arumeria 14, 31, 32, 87
        That Sounds Good Jazz Pension 16, 31, 90, 91
    Ryokans (Traditional Inns) 3, 15, 31
        Youth Hostel Murataya Ryokan 32
    Youth Hostels 3, 15, 31
        Nikko Suginamiki Youth Hostel 30, 31, 91, 92
        Youth Hostel Kurashaki 16
        Youth Hostel Murataya Ryokan 16
Adaptors (Power) 106
Adzuki (Red Beans) 11, 74, 75
Airbnbs See Accommodation
Alcoholic Drinks 63
    Beer 11, 39, 47, 79, 106
        Asahi Factory 79
        Beer Festivals 51, 79
    Sake (Rice Wine) 3, 46, 47, 75, 78, 79, 103, 106
        Imaya Tsukasa Sake Brewery 78
        Jumai-Daiginjo-Shu 79
        New Sake 79, 80
        Premium Sake 79
        Sake Breweries 79
        Sake Cups 79
        Sake Museum 79
        Sake Town 79
        Sparkling Sake 46, 78, 79
        Table Sake 79
    Spirits 3, 47, 63, 79, 106
        Awamori 79, 103
        Masahiro Awamori Brewery 80
        Gin and Tonic 27, 79, 83
        Highballs 27
        Shochu 47, 79, 103, 106
        Vodka 27, 79
        Whiskey 27, 79
    Wine 3, 47, 63, 79, 106
        Argentinian 79
        Australian 79
        Chilean 79
        Ikeda Wine Castle 78, 79
        Wine Research 79
Ambulance 106
Andy Warhol 27
Aquaria 51
    Umitamago Aquarium 51
Art Galleries See Museums & Art Galleries
Art Islands See SHIKOKU, Naoshima
Australian Department of Foreign Affairs 106
Autumn Foliage 106
Awamori See Alcoholic Drinks, Spirits

B

Bakeries 39, 63, 75
Barbecue See Restaurants
Barley 11, 19, 63, 79
Bars 80

Beer See Alcoholic Drinks
Bento Boxes 43, 95
    Eki Bento 43, 44
Botanic Gardens 51
    Ritsurin Garden 95
Bread 11, 15, 27, 43, 103
Breakfasts 3, 15, 16, 18, 19, 27, 28, 31, 43, 58, 59, 87
    Buffet 15, 27, 28, 59
    Continental 15, 27
Broth 91
Buckwheat 11, 23, 35, 75, 79, 90, 91

C

Cakes 3, 11, 43, 75, 76, 103
    Chiffon Cakes 75
    Ishimura 75
    Kutchen 74, 75
    Otaco 75
    Taiyaki 51
Car Hire 19, 106
Ceramic Dolls 99
Cereals 27
Cheese 19, 47
Cherry Blossom 27, 106
Chicken See Meat
Child Kitchen 23
Chilli Sauce 60
Chocolate 3, 47, 63, 83
    Chocolate Coated Bananas 51
    Hot Chocolate 83
Christmas 51
Clothes 106
Coconut 59
Coeliac Disease 7, 11, 35, 71, 79
    Australia and New Zealand 11
    China and Japan 11
    Diagnosis 11
Coeliac Travel Website 8
Coffee See Drinks (Non-Alcoholic)
Confectionery 11
Convenience Stores (Konbini) 3, 19, 43, 47, 75, 78, 79, 83, 106, 107
    Aeon Mini 43
    Family Mart 43
    Lawson Station 43, 75, 83
    Seven Eleven 43, 83
Cookies 75
Cooking 3, 15, 55
Cooking Classes 3, 22, 23
Cooking Utensils 55
    Cooking Chopsticks 55
    Silicon Cups 71
Credit Cards 63, 106
Crockery 3, 31, 55
    Cups 55
    Glasses 31, 55
    Plates 31, 55
Currency 106
    Yen 106
Curries 30, 39, 87
Cutlery 3, 31, 55
    Forks 31
    Knives 31, 55
    Spoons 31, 55

D

Dairy 3, 63, 71
    Butter 71
    Cheese 63, 71
    Cream 71
    Custard 75
    Icecream 3, 51, 71, 75

Gelatos 39
Lady Borden 75
Magnums 71, 75
MOW 71, 75
NorgenVass 75
Rhubarb-Haskap 75
Milk 71
Soy See Soy
Yoghurt 27, 58, 59, 71, 75, 82, 83, 87

Data 106

Day Tours 19

Degustation 95

Department Stores 3, 12, 43, 63, 64, 66, 67, 99, 106
Iwataya 64, 66

Desserts 3, 39, 75, 82, 86, 87
Creme Caramels 75
Godiva 75, 83
Icecream See Dairy
Rice Puddings 75
Zenzai 74, 75

Dietary Requirements 3, 19, 87

Dinners 3, 14, 15, 19, 27, 31, 39, 43, 46, 59, 87

Donburi (Rice Bowls) 11, 35, 43

Dosages 107

Drinks 43
Vending Machine 84

Drinks (Alcoholic) See Alcoholic Drinks

Drinks (Non-Alcoholic) 63, 83
Coffee 3, 63, 83
Coffee Shops 83
Drip Coffee Bags 83, 107
Filtered Coffee 83
Lavazza 83
Low Sugar Drinks 83
Mixer Drinks 83
No Sugar 83
Tea 63, 83
Green Tea 82, 83
Matcha 58, 59, 75, 83
Tea Ceremony 83, 84
Tonic Water 83
Unsweetened 83
Yoghurt Drinks 83

Driving 106

Dry Ice Machine 63

Dumplings 23, 99

E

Earthquakes 106

Eggs 3, 10, 27, 35, 43, 47, 51, 59, 60, 62, 63, 71, 72, 91
Egg Vending Machine 63
Omelettes 11, 43, 58, 59, 67, 71

Eki Bento See Bento Boxes

Emergency Phone Numbers 106

Entertainment 106

Etiquette 106

Events 3, 51, 106
Triennale 95

F

Fake Food 34, 35
Fake Food Workshop Riki 22

Festivals 3, 27, 51, 76, 106
Beer Festivals See Alcoholic Drinks, Beer
Flower Festivals 51
Hojoya Festival 51, 52
Naked Man Festival 51
O-Bon 106
Sanja Matsuri Festival 51

Fire 106

Fish See Seafood

Flour 10, 15, 59, 63, 64, 71
Chick-Pea 39
Potato Flour 99

Fruit 3, 11, 19, 27, 59, 63, 67, 95, 103

Apples 67
Avocados 103
Bananas 59, 63, 75, 76
Bankan 67, 95
Blood Oranges 58
Blueberries 67
Cherries 67
Chestnuts 67, 75
Citrus 67, 95, 96
Coconut 58, 63
Figs 59
Fruit Drinks 103
Fruit Juices 27, 63
Gingko 75
Grapes 67, 71, 79
Guavas 83
Horse Chestnuts 75
Jellied Fruit 71, 75
Kiwi Fruit 67
Lemons 95
Mandarins (Mekan) 63, 66, 67, 75, 95
Mangoes 67, 75
Mikans See Mandarins
Musk Melons 67, 75
Nectarines 71
Oranges 95
Passionfruit 67
Peaches 67
Pears 67, 71
Persimmons 68, 75
Pineapples 67, 83
Plums 67
Picked Plums 47
Rock Melons 75
Strawberries 59, 63, 67, 75
Sultanas 47, 58, 59
Tangerines 95
Yuzu 67, 95

Furukawa Cooking School 22, 23

Futons 31

G

Garbage 106

Genetics 11

Gluten-Free Highlights
Hokkaido 87
Honshu 91
Kyushu 99
Okinawa 103
Shikoku 95

Google Maps 106

Google Translate 7, 15, 19, 63, 106, 107

Green Grocers 67, 68

Growers' Market 3, 48, 62, 63, 67, 68

Guest Houses See Accommodation

Gyoza 23

H

Habu (Snake) 79, 80

Hanami 27

HOKKAIDO 15, 27, 28, 31, 47, 67, 71, 75, 78, 79, 87
Gluten-Free Highlights 87
Hakodate 42
Ikeda 75
Happiness Dairy 75
Kamoenai 28
Kiritappu coast 87
Kushiro 3, 30, 35, 87
Niseko 3, 75, 87
Rausu 26, 87
Rebun Island 15
Sapporo 3, 31, 38, 42, 51, 54, 71, 87
Former Government Building 87
Susukino 38
Shiretoko 87
Wakkanai 3, 14, 31, 32, 87

HONSHU 15, 27
Daizen 100% soba restaurant 90, 91
Gluten-Free Highlights 91
Hakone 31, 51
Hiroshima 31, 75, 79

109

Ise 34
Koguchi 18
Kumano-Kodo Pilgrimage 18, 20, 68
Kurashiki 16, 34, 35
Kyoto 31, 38, 70
Mine 27
Nagano 3, 23, 75, 90, 91
Nakasendo Way 18, 19, 20
   Shinchaya 19
   Takahara 68
Niigata 78, 79
Nikko 3, 82, 83, 91
Okayama 51
Osaka 15
Saijo 75, 79
Sakaiminato 56
Sekigahara 20
Takayama 3, 31, 50, 51, 91, 92
Tateyama 83
Tazawako 3, 6, 16, 31, 90
Tokyo 12, 31, 39, 51, 62, 70, 75, 76, 83, 84, 91
   Asakusa 75, 76
   Omiya 35, 91, 92
   Roppongi Hills 74, 75
   Saitama 3, 90, 91
   Tokyo Station 107
Tsuruoka 14, 82
Tsuwano 26

Hostels See Accommodation

Hotels See Accommodation

Hot-Pots (Nabe, Shabu-Shabu) 3, 11, 20, 23, 26, 27, 35, 71, 87, 90, 91, 103, 104

Hundred-Yen Shop 55

I

IC Cards 107
   Icoca 107
   Nimoca 107
   Suica 107
Ice Machine 63
Ice Packs 63
Ingredients 3, 8, 63, 75
International Driver's Licence 106
Internet 106
Itinerary 15

J

Jam 58, 59
Japan Rail Passes 106

K

Kaldi Coffee Farm 12, 47, 59, 63, 79
Kanji 7
Kentucky Fried Chicken 51
Kitchen Appliances 31, 55
   Cooktop 55
   Electric Jug 27, 31, 55
   Hotplate 31
   Microwave 27, 31, 55, 63
   Oven 55
   Refrigerator 27, 31, 55
   Toaster 55
Kitchen Utensils
   Chopping Board 55
   Colander 55
   Egg Slice 55
   Frying Pan 31, 55
   Mixing Bowl 55
   Pots & Pans 3, 55
   Rice Cooker 55
   Saucepans 31, 55
Koji Mold 79
Konbini See Convenience Stores
Konbu (Kelp) See Seaweeds
Kumano-Kodo Pilgrimage See HONSHU
Kyoto 11, 15, 39
KYUSHU 63, 67, 76, 99, 107
   Aso Town 3, 72, 80, 99, 100
   Beppu 51, 74, 75
   Fukuoka 3, 15, 23, 38, 40, 50, 51, 52, 55, 63, 66, 70, 72, 75, 79, 80, 83, 98, 99, 100
      Hakata 99
      Ijiri 68
      Ōhashi 22, 23, 63, 66
      River Naka 99
      Tenjin 12, 98, 99, 100
      Gluten-Free Highlights 99
   Kagoshima 3, 42, 99
   Kumamoto 42
   Mount Aso 99
   Nagasaki 47, 66
   Takamori 16, 32
   Yakushima 3, 98, 99
      Anbo 98, 99

L

Language 7, 107
Language School 15
Lonely Planet 15
Luggage 107
   Luggage Forwarding 107
Lunches 3, 19, 27, 39, 43, 59, 60
   Buffet 19, 51, 87
   Hotels 19
   Picnics 19, 63

M

Macdonalds 11
Map 105
Meat 3, 23, 35, 43, 59, 63, 67, 70, 71, 91
   Beef 71
   Chicken 35, 39, 43, 47, 51, 63, 87, 103
      Charcoal Chicken 35, 95
      Chicken Karaage 59, 91
      Chicken Sashimi 35
      Yakitori 11, 43, 51, 52, 70
   Duck 87
   Lamb 51, 71
   Pork 71
      Ham 87
      Spam 39, 71, 103
   Steak 35
   Whale 35
Medical 107
   Hospitals 107
   Medical History 107
   Medicines 107
Medicine Caterpillar 87
Miso (Fermented Soybeans) 11, 18, 103
   Miso Soup 11, 14, 27, 58, 59
Mobile Phone 107
Mobile Wi-Fi 106
Mochi (Sweet Rice Balls) 3, 10, 11, 47, 51, 63, 75
   Icecream Mochi 75
   Strawberry Mochi 95
Museums & Art Galleries 51
   Benesse House Museum 27
   Hakone Outdoor Sculpture Museum 51
   Museum Restaurant Issen 27
   National Museum of Art 51
   Okurayama Ski Jump & Winter Sports Museum 51
   Sapporo Art Museum 51
   Soba Museum 75
   Tonkururen Togakushi Soba Museum 23
   Volcano Museum 99

N

Nabe See Hot-Pots (Nabe, Shabu-Shabu)
Nakasendo Way See HONSHU
Naoshima See SHIKOKU
New Year 27, 51, 52, 103
Nibbles See Snacks
Noodles 3, 11, 19, 23, 35, 39, 43, 59, 63, 71, 91, 99, 103
   Ramen 11, 23, 103
   Soba 11, 23, 24, 35, 75, 90, 91

Udon 11, 99
Nuts 47, 63
　Cashews 47
　Macadamias 47
　Peanuts 47

O

Oats 11, 19, 63
OKINAWA 15, 39, 47, 48, 52, 62, 63, 66, 67, 68, 71, 79, 99, 102, 104
　Gluten-Free Highlights 103
　Itoman 3, 62, 63, 67, 68, 70, 103, 104
　　AAA (SanA) Shopping Centre 103
　　Itoman Fish Centre 102, 103
　Naha 3, 102, 103
　Yaeyama Islands 15, 83, 103
　　Ishigaki 3, 103
Okinomiyaki (Cabbage Pancake) 51, 59, 60
Omelettes See Eggs
Omiyage (Souvenirs) 11, 19, 75, 76
Onigiri (Rice Balls) 43, 46, 47, 63, 91
Onsens (Hot Springs) 31, 67, 107
Orange Train 67
Orchards 67
Oyakodon (Chicken & Egg Rice Bowl) 59

P

Paella 38, 39, 59
Pancakes 59, 63, 91
Pasta 27, 39, 43
　Fettucinne 103
　Spaghetti 59, 103
　Vermicelli 23
Pensions See Accommodation
Pharmacy 107
Phone Cards 107
Pickles 10, 11, 27, 35, 43, 58, 59, 67
Pizza 27, 39
Planning 15
Police 106
Porridge 87
Potato Chips 47, 99
Practical Tips & Advice 3
Public Holidays 106
　Golden Week 27, 106
Public Phones 107

R

Railway Stations 3, 27, 35, 43, 83, 99
　Railway Station Signage 107
Ready-Made Meals 63
Recycling 106
Restaurant Cards 7, 8, 15, 35
Restaurants 3, 11, 19, 27, 35, 51, 59, 90, 99, 106
　Barbecue 3, 35, 36, 51, 71
　　Gyu-kaku 35
　　Robata 35
　Cafe Yukiya 86, 87
　French 39
　Hamazushi 35, 36
　Indian 3, 39, 40
　Italian 3, 39
　Izakaya 3, 35
　Japanese 79
　Mexican 38, 39
　Nepalese 39
　Sanzoku Tabiji Restaurant 98, 99
　Spanish 3, 38, 39
　Starbucks 83
　Sushi Isogai Restaurant 12, 98, 99
　Suttu's Restaurant Kagra 87
　Tapas Bars 38, 39
　Teishoku 3, 35

Thai 3, 38, 39
Tonden 87, 88
Tsuruga 87
Yakiniku 35
Yakitori 34
Yayoiken 34, 35
Rice 23, 27, 34, 35, 43, 47, 58, 59, 63, 79
　Fried Rice 59
　Instant Rice 63
　Kettle Steamed Rice 95
　Pickle Rice 98, 99
　Pounded Rice Sticks 51
　Rice Paper Rolls 23, 60, 63
　Rice Polishing Machine 63
　Rice Vinegar 22, 23
Rice Crackers 11, 19, 47
　Class 23
Rice Paper Rolls 59
Roaming Charges 107
Romaji 107
Rye 11, 19, 63
Ryokans See Accommodation

S

Safety Tips 106
Saitama See Honshu, Tokyo
Sake See Alcoholic Drinks
Salads 27, 35, 39, 42, 59, 67, 91
　Potato Salad 43
　Pumpkin Salad 43
Sandwiches 43
Sapporo See HOKKAIDO
Sashimi 11, 12, 23, 35, 42, 43, 51, 59, 71, 99
　Seared Bonito Sashimi 95, 96
Seafood 3, 35, 39, 63, 71, 87, 91, 95, 102, 103
　Clams 59, 87
　Crabs 71
　　Hairy Crab 87
　　King Crab 87
　Fish 23, 27, 34, 58, 71, 87
　　Blowfish 18, 35, 71
　　Carpacchio 23
　　Eel 11
　　Fish Markets 51
　　Fish Patties 43, 63, 70, 71
　　Flounder 87
　　Flying Fish 71, 87, 98
　　John Dory 99
　　Karei 87
　　Miso Fish 95, 96
　　Salmon 47, 59
　　Salmon Roe 47, 87
　　Salt-Grilled 10
　　Seared Bonito (Katsuo no Tataki) 95
　　Swordfish 58
　　Tuna 47
　Lobsters 103
　Octopus 51, 71, 87
　　Octopus Gills 87
　　Octopus Head 87
　Oysters 91
　Prawns & Shrimp 47, 59, 60, 71, 87
　Scallops 12, 14, 87, 103
　Sea Cucumbers 71, 87
　Seafood Markets 71
　　Nijo Fish Market 71
　Sea Urchin Roe 87
　Squid 87, 103
　Tunicates 71
　Whelks 71, 87
Seaweeds 47, 59, 87
　Kelp (Konbu) 87, 88
　　Exhibition 87
　Nori 47
　Wakame 67
Seniors Discounts 107
Shabu-Shabu See Hot-Pots (Nabe, Shabu-Shabu)
SHIKOKU 15, 27, 67, 95
　Art Islands 27, 95

111

    Naoshima 3, 27, 94, 95
    Teshima 66, 95
  Cape Ashizuri 95
  Cape Muroto 95
  Gluten-Free Highlights 95
  Kochi 3, 95
    Kochi Sunday Market 67, 95, 96
  Matsuyama 3, 95
    Matsuyama Castle 95
    Mitsu 95
    Mitsu Market 95
  Sukumo 3, 95, 96
  Takamatsu 46, 76, 95
  Uchiko 3, 95, 96
Shinkansen 43, 44, 92, 99, 107
Shochu See Alcoholic Drinks, Spirits
SIM Cards 107
Slippers 31
Smoking 35
Snacks 3, 18, 19, 43, 46, 47, 63, 103
  Nibbles 43
  Rice Crackers 24
Snow 107
Soba See Noodles
Soy
  Soy Beans See Vegetables, Edamame
  Soy Milk 35, 91, 103, 104
  Soy Sauce 11, 12, 15, 18, 19, 23, 35, 51, 59, 63, 64, 67, 71, 103
  Soy Yoghurt 87
  Tofu 3, 59, 63, 67, 70, 71, 75, 103
  Tofuyo 79, 102, 103
  Yuba 31, 91
Soyjoy Bars 10, 11, 19, 47, 48, 63
Soy Sauce See Soy
Spirits See Alcoholic Drinks
Sports 106
Stir Fries 59, 60, 71
Storage Lockers 106, 107
Street Food 3, 51
  Takoyaki 51
  Yatai 50
Sugidama (Cedar Twig Balls) 79
Suito 23
Sumo 51
Supermarkets 3, 7, 10, 11, 19, 31, 42, 43, 46, 47, 48, 59, 62, 63, 70, 71, 75, 79, 83, 103, 106, 107
Super Ring 99
Sushi 3, 11, 19, 23, 24, 35, 42, 43, 51, 59, 71, 91, 92, 95
  Classes 8, 23
  Inakazushi 95
  Seared Bonito 43
  Vegetarian 43
Sweetfish 50, 51
Sweets 3, 43, 75

T

Tacos 59, 63
  Taco Rice 39, 59, 102, 103
  Taco Sauce 63
Takeaways 3, 27, 43, 63, 95
Tamari 63
Tatami 31
Tattoos 107
Tazawako See HONSHU
Tea See Drinks (Non-Alcoholic)
Tempura 11, 43
Tofu See Soy
Tofuyo See Soy
Tokyo See HONSHU
Tour Company 15, 19
Tours & Treks 3, 19, 79

Transport 106
Travel Insurance 107
Tsunamis 106
Typhoons 15, 107

U

Utensils 55

V

Vegemite 15
Vegetables 3, 11, 23, 35, 39, 43, 47, 51, 58, 59, 63, 64, 67, 71, 87, 91, 95, 103
  Bean Sprouts 67, 68
  Bitter Melon 67
  Cabbage 59
  Capsicums 59
  Carrots 47, 59, 67
  Corn 51
  Daikon 87
  Edamame (Soy Beans) 43, 47, 91
  Eggplant 66
  Ginger 60
  Leeks 8, 103
  Lettuce 59
  Micro-Greens 59, 67
  Mountain Vegetables 91
  Mushrooms 59, 66, 67, 87
    Enokitake 67
    Shitake 67
  Okra 87
  Onions 59
  Potatoes 51, 75, 83, 103
  Pumpkin 75
  Purple Vegetables 103
  Sprouts 59, 67
  Sweet Potatoes 47, 67, 79, 82, 83, 95
    Beni-Imo (Purple Sweet Potatoes) 39, 48, 67, 103
    Hot Sweet Potatoes 46
    Sweet Potato Slab 96
  Tomatoes 47, 59, 67
  Vegetable Dumpling Soup 99
  Vegetable Patties 43
  Vegetable Snacks 48
Vending Machines 27, 78, 84, 107
Venues 3, 51
Vinegar 11
Visas
  Toursit Visa 107
Voltage 106

W

Wagashi 75
Wagashi (Sweets) 83
Walks 3, 19
Waste Disposal 55
Water 107
Weather 107
Wheat 6, 7, 11, 19, 23, 35, 51, 63, 75, 99
Wi-Fi 106
Wine See Alcoholic Drinks
Winter Olympics 91

Y

Yaeyama Islands See OKINAWA
Yakitori See also Restaurants; See Meat, Chicken
Yakushima See KYUSHU
Yatsuhoshi 11
Yoghurt See Dairy
Youth Hostels See Accommodation
Yukata 31

Z

Zenzai See Desserts

www.ingramcontent.com/pod-product-compliance
Lightning Source LLC
Chambersburg PA
CBHW051617030426
42334CB00030B/3233